Developing Communication Skills for Veterinary Practice

Jane R. Shaw, DVM, PhD
Professor
Department of Clinical Sciences
College of Veterinary Medicine and Biomedical Sciences
Colorado State University
Fort Collins, Colorado, USA

Jason B. Coe, DVM, PhD
Professor
Department of Population Medicine
Ontario Veterinary College
University of Guelph
Guelph, Ontario, Canada

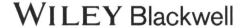
WILEY Blackwell

Library of Congress Cataloging-in-Publication Data

Names: Shaw, Jane R., author. | Coe, Jason B. (Jason Bradley), author.
Title: Developing communication skills for veterinary practice / Jane R.
  Shaw, Jason B. Coe.
Description: Hoboken, NJ : Wiley-Blackwell 2023. | Includes bibliographical
  references and index.
Identifiers: LCCN 2022059959 (print) | LCCN 2022059960 (ebook) | ISBN
  9781119382713 (paperback) | ISBN 9781119382720 (adobe pdf) | ISBN
  9781119382751 (epub)
Subjects: MESH: Veterinary Medicine–methods | Communication |
  Professional-Patient Relations
Classification: LCC SF610.5 (print) | LCC SF610.5 (ebook) | NLM SF 610.5 |
  DDC 636.089–dc23/eng/20230323
LC record available at https://lccn.loc.gov/2022059959
LC ebook record available at https://lccn.loc.gov/2022059960

Cover Design: Wiley
Cover Images: © kali9/Getty Images; Pressmaster/Shutterstock; Juice Flair/Shutterstock;
Seventyfour/Adobe Stock Photos

Set in 9.5/12.5pt STIXTwoText by Straive, Pondicherry, India
Printed and bound by CPI Group (UK) Ltd, Croydon, CR0 4YY
C9781119382713_180324

We dedicate this book to our parents.

Evelyn and Donald Shaw provided me with every opportunity and endless love and support to follow my dreams of becoming a veterinarian. ~ JRS

Bruce and Frances Coe, to whose absolute support I owe everything. ~ JBC

Contents

About the Authors

Neither of us knew when we first met in 1999 that two-and-a-half decades later, we would be writing a book together on veterinary communication. At the time of our first meeting, Jane Shaw was a graduate student enrolled in the Department of Population Medicine at the University of Guelph with a veterinary degree from Michigan State University, and Jason Coe was a third-year student veterinarian at the Ontario Veterinary College (OVC), University of Guelph. We met fortuitously one Saturday morning in OVC's Veterinary Teaching Hospital Wellness Clinic, a student-centered primary care service, where Jane was practicing, teaching, and supervising students, and Jason was volunteering to gain more clinical experience prior to graduation.

With a focus on clinical communication, we both completed doctorates in veterinary epidemiology under Cindy Adams, MSW, PhD, who implemented the first veterinary communication curriculum in North America at OVC. In addition, we spent time in clinical practice, which informs our teaching and research in veterinary communication. Jane spent 10 years in academic and private practice in companion animal medicine, whereas Jason's 9 years of clinical experience were rooted in mixed animal followed by food animal practice.

We also have decades of experience as dedicated educators, teaching students in two of the leading veterinary communication programs in North America. In these roles, we continue to develop skills-based, learner-centered clinical communication curricula, which received commendations from the American Veterinary Medical Association Council on Education for innovation. We are committed to student veterinarians' and, more broadly, veterinary professionals' success in practice by **equipping them with a toolbox of communication skills** to manage both routine and challenging client and team conversations. The result is reflected in positive alumni ratings of our programs and the career performance and testimonials of our graduates.

As leaders in the field, we often venture out of the classroom to speak nationally and internationally to veterinary professionals at conferences and continuing-education events. We participate in and offer intensive interactive communication workshops with strong reputations for **transforming the practice of veterinary medicine**. We coach veterinary professionals in their examination rooms as they communicate with their clients and care for their patients. Through these experiences, we are privileged to witness individuals and entire practice teams taking their communication skills to the next level. Veterinary professionals reap benefits in the form of increased practice performance, client satisfaction, client adherence, patient health, and career fulfillment.

In addition to teaching and coaching, a significant component of our professional identities is developing and conducting evidence-based research in veterinary communication. As trained epidemiologists, we implement research in the field, often video-recording client interactions in veterinary practices and interviewing key informants, including veterinary professionals and their clients. In writing this book, we **translate our research findings into hands-on recommendations** to enhance interactions in veterinary practice. In all these endeavors, we maintain a pragmatic view where we strive to be practical, skills-focused, and outcome-based. In doing so, we hope to enhance uptake of new approaches, change habits, and maximize results.

In veterinary practice, much meaning stems from day-to-day conversations with veterinary team members and clients. **Veterinary professionals empowered with communication tools enjoy more satisfying interactions and relationships** and affirmation of their day-to-day work in veterinary medicine. And when discussions do go awry, as they will, veterinary professionals with the skills and capabilities to manage difficult conversations experience less stress and derive more fulfillment.

For 25 years, we took note of what we learned individually and together and packaged it up for you. This book offers proven methods that withstood the test of time in academic and clinical settings among diverse veterinary professionals. Now it's your turn. Are you curious to see where the rubber meets the road in your interactions? If so, throughout this book, we help you develop your communication toolbox to enhance your daily exchanges with clients, colleagues, and beyond.

How to Use This Book

We would like to begin by sharing our underlying intentions for developing this communication resource and by highlighting a number of unique aspects of the book. We strove for this book to be user-friendly, accessible, practical, and applicable to all members of the veterinary team. We hope the book is used as a communication skills operating manual; we expect the cover to become coffee-stained, sections to be highlighted and underlined throughout, and pages to be marked and dog-eared.

The book is organized into tasks of the **clinical appointment,** with chapters flowing from opening-the-interaction, information-gathering, and attending to relationships and tasks to diagnostic and treatment planning, and closing-the-interaction. In each chapter, we showcase key communication skills integral to achieving these tasks. We define the communication skill, demonstrate techniques, and provide examples. Over the course of the book, we introduce a **communication toolbox** including 20 communication skills.

We emphasize the importance of **effective communication with clients and colleagues**. In each chapter, we present routine and challenging scenarios in day-to-day practice, and we model how to use the communication skills in both caregiver and collegial interactions. How you communicate with your clients is the bread and butter of your business and establishes long-term client relationships and a strong client base. How you communicate with your colleagues defines the veterinary practice culture, which is integral to creating a healthy, functional workplace environment in which employees thrive.

At the end of each chapter, we offer **learning activities** to work through, individually or collaboratively, in a small group or with the entire practice team. Through these exercises, we outline a developmental curriculum to build a strong communication toolbox. The book provides ample opportunities to practice the communication skills through either a self-led or guided experiential learning process. The tasks progress from easier, structured, low-risk approaches (e.g. skill spotting exercises, guided reflections, and individual role-play) to more challenging, small-group, high-stakes methods (e.g. in-the-moment coaching or communication and video-review rounds). Over time, the focus shifts from personal communication skill development to coaching and mentoring colleagues.

One key takeaway is that the **communication toolbox is transferable** to all areas of veterinary practice, to any career path, and to one's own personal life. Although this book is situated in companion animal primary care, the communication tools are critical to success and fulfillment in both general and specialty practices, and in equine, livestock, avian, exotic, zoo, and wildlife medicine. They are equally important for working in laboratory medicine, governmental and non-governmental agencies, public health, regulatory medicine, and industry – not to mention supporting the inter- and intra-professional communication that is instrumental in the referral DVM-specialist relationship, as well as in developing partnerships with vendors, behaviorists, groomers, doggie daycare providers, breeders, and crematorium directors. Finally, these are life skills, and they work well with spouses, partners, children, other family members, and neighbors and at book clubs, on ballfields, or in volunteer organizations.

We take into consideration the **myriad of ways in which we communicate** with our clients and colleagues. Face-to-face interactions still predominate, followed by telephone and then electronic communication (e.g. email or text) or virtual care. Each method has its own purpose and special considerations and can be highly effective in getting a message across. Unfortunately, if used inappropriately, each modality can result in miscommunication and challenges.

Furthermore, we weave in aspects of technology that can enhance or detract from communication. As with any tool, technology has its time and place. It is critical to know when and how to use each type, from the telephone, whiteboards, and printed care instructions to treatment plans sent via email, or interactive video consultations. In the "Talk through Technology" section of each chapter, we outline best practices for **complementary use of technology**.

As leading researchers in veterinary communication, we also share **Research Spotlights** that highlight relevant findings from our veterinary communication studies. Two strong evidence-based books, one on medical communication (Silverman et al. 2013) and the other on veterinary communication (Adams and Kurtz 2017), provide a more thorough and extensive review of the broader clinical-communication literature. Our emphasis is on translating our research into practice – how to apply the findings to real-life scenarios that will inform and enhance client and colleague interactions, develop the veterinary practice, and further veterinary careers.

Here are our **12 recommendations** for how to get the most out of this book:

1. **Capitalize on strengths.** Be aware of your communication assets on the table. Know what they are and how they work. Then use this book to fine-tune, dust off, or sharpen communication skills that may be currently underutilized.
2. **Stretch outside your comfort zone.** Try on the communication skills, even if they do not "fit" at first. Start with learning the stem phrases, then implement the scripted examples, and, finally, improvise and own the skills. It may feel fake or artificial at first; however, with continued application and adaption of the skills to fit individual styles, over time the skills will feel natural, authentic, and genuine.
3. **Be forgiving, and let go of perfection.** Practice makes better, not perfect. Communication competency has a high ceiling, like many other clinical skills – clinical reasoning, surgery, or interpreting test results. Strive to be a good communicator, know that mistakes will be made, and make a recovery when it does not go as liked. The resulting relationship is often stronger after repairing a mishap.
4. **Self-reflect, and be courageous.** Be fearless, vulnerable, and open to taking a good hard look at the current communication skills in your toolbox. Regrettably, our perceptions of our communication competence are far from accurate. So, self-reflect on client and colleague interactions, and be bold and request feedback from mentors and peers to identify blind spots.
5. **Engage with this book.** Each chapter includes a traditional knowledge component to foster awareness and understanding of communication concepts. And an interactive section with learning exercises that provide opportunities to practice the skills, identify strengths and challenges, and set learning goals for continued development.
6. **Keep a journal, and document progress.** Before embarking, start a communication journal to capture insights, lessons learned, and communication goals and to mark growth, progress, and milestones. Look back in the pages to see the headway made and be accountable for achieving objectives.
7. **Apply the skills with clients and colleagues**. Use these communication skills to transform day-to-day client interactions, address challenging conversations, and lend a compassionate ear to clients. Do the very same thing with colleagues to create a veterinary team culture characterized by strong communication, morale, teamwork, and retention. Enhance self-esteem and confidence. Enjoy going to work. And make a difference in the lives of colleagues, clients, and patients.
8. **Read this book multiple times with different intents**. For example, on the first read, work on building your communication skills toolbox. Then, the second time, lead your team or veterinary practice through the exercises, developing their skills and coaching techniques. On the

third read, mentor others on the practice team while they coach their colleagues. The goal is to create a critical mass of individuals to build, lead, and sustain a communicative and collaborative team culture.

9. **Teach the team the communication skills.** It takes a village in a veterinary practice to serve clients and care for patients. Set colleagues up for success by equipping them with the communication skills they need to excel in their positions. Set the practice up for success by expanding the team of effective communicators and delegating appropriate conversations (e.g. agenda-setting, preventive care education, follow-up progress calls, or sharing diagnostic test results).

10. **Be creative in involving the team**. Depending on the personality, character, and culture of the team, make it fun by designing communication role-plays, *Jeopardy*, or "choose your own adventure." Or, as the team implements skills, set goals, assess metrics, and monitor trends, such as changes in appointment efficiency, veterinarian average client transaction, or client reviews. Ask teammates who model exemplary communication skills to mentor and coach colleagues.

11. **Get a leg up or a new lease on practice.** For new employees or early-career veterinary graduates, the communication skills ease the professional transition. Entering with a well-equipped communication toolbox promotes victories and reduces failures associated with trial and error. For late-career veterinary professionals, these communication skills reignite and reinvigorate "the why" – to enjoy meaningful interactions with colleagues and clients and to care for patients.

12. **Take the communication skills home.** Use these communication skills when interacting with clients, colleagues, family members, neighbors, and friends, and see how they change life in and outside the veterinary practice. Reap the rewards in client and collegial interactions, as well as in family and social life, leading to more fulfilling conversations and deeper connections.

Suggested Timeline

To set realistic expectations and maintain momentum, we suggest the following timeline as guidance for how long it will take to complete each chapter and the associated learning exercises individually or as a practice team:

1. Chapter 1 – Introduction – 1 week
2. Chapter 2 – Communication Styles – 3 weeks
3. Chapter 3 – Opening-the-Interaction – 2 weeks
4. Chapter 4 – Information-Gathering – 6 weeks
5. Chapter 5 – Attending to Relationships – 3 weeks
6. Chapter 6 – Attending to Tasks – 3 weeks
7. Chapter 7 – Diagnostic and Treatment Planning – 8 weeks
8. Chapter 8 – Closing-the-interaction – 2 weeks
9. Chapter 9 – Communication Coaching – 6 weeks
10. Chapter 10 – Transferring the Skills to Various Contexts – 2 weeks
11. Chapter 11 – Now What? – 2 weeks

   Total: 38 Weeks – Approximately 9 months

References

Adams, C.L. and Kurtz, S. (2017). *Skills for Communicating in Veterinary Medicine*. Parsippany, NJ. Dewpoint Publishing.

Silverman, J., Kurtz, S., and Draper, J. (2013). *Skills for Communicating with Patients*. London, England. CRC Press.

Acknowledgments

This book is the culmination of decades of trials and tribulations and collaborations and contributions. First, we thank our mentors in veterinary medicine, Dr. Cindy Adams and Dr. Brenda Bonnett, and colleagues in human medicine Dr. Suzanne Kurtz and Dr. Debra Roter; they are pioneers in their fields and laid a rigorous foundation. Second, we are grateful to all the student veterinarians, graduate students, simulated clients, communication coaches, coordinators, and co-instructors we worked with through the years. They taught us more than we taught them and left lasting fingerprints on our knowledge and programs. Third, we recognize the support and advocacy provided by our colleges, deans, associate deans, and department heads, who envisioned the future, invested, and committed to equipping veterinarians with communication skills for success. Finally, many veterinary clinics opened their doors, hearts, and minds to participate in live learning laboratories to put our teachings into practice.

Specifically, we appreciate individual contributions to this book. We are indebted to Dr. Susan Ring deRosset, who served as our editor. Her combined veterinary and literary background provided instrumental suggestions that shaped this book. Courtney Hensel contributed to formatting and layout; Maddi Funk created the figures; Catherine Groves assisted with final edits; Dr. Naomi Nishi who provided counsel on justice, equity, diversity, and inclusion; and Dr. Tracey Jensen, Dr. Elizabeth Alvarez, and Lorna Wyllsun reviewed early versions of chapters and provided feedback.

And far from last, our families who nurtured us in becoming and supported us as veterinarians and academicians; it would not have been possible without their unconditional love and care. The support of friends and social outings and adventures provided respite and fueled creativity. Our own companion animals provided unconditional love, poignant life lessons, and lived meaning of the human-animal bond.

1

Introduction

Abstract

In this chapter, we lay the groundwork for why it is worth investing in developing a strong communication toolbox consisting of 20 communication skills with proven success. We begin with recognizing that communication skill-building takes practice and time. Then we argue that communication is both a science and an art. The science of communication entails using the skills with purpose and intention. The art of communication requires using the skills adeptly not only in straightforward interactions but also in nuanced, complex, challenging, and high-stakes situations with diverse individuals. We acknowledge the stressful context of a busy veterinary practice and the daily challenge of attending to tasks (i.e. getting work done) and relationships (i.e. building trust with clients and colleagues). Being successful and striving for the right balance requires establishing long-term relationships with clients and colleagues. And we emphasize that team communication makes the difference between a healthy practice environment and a dysfunctional one. We conclude that embracing both roles – as animal healthcare experts as well as partners to our clients and colleagues – promotes positive outcomes for the veterinary practice and our colleagues, clients, patients, and, importantly, ourselves.

SELF-ASSESSMENT QUESTIONS (True or False) See the end of the chapter for the answer key.

1. Effective communication can be learned through practice, feedback, and coaching.
2. Effective communication is critical to achieving significant outcomes for the veterinary practice; with colleagues, clients, and patients; and self.
3. Effective communication is integral to maintaining and sustaining a healthy practice culture and interprofessional relationships.
4. Effective communication takes more time.

Communication Matters

Communication is the most common clinical procedure performed daily in veterinary practice and prevails in every client and colleague interaction. For client service coordinators specifically, their entire day is spent communicating with others. A veterinary professional involved in 20 appointments per day will engage in more than 200,000 client interactions over a 40-year career

(Shaw et al. 2012). This does not account for the too-numerous-to-count colleague-to-colleague conversations. The final sum is an astounding number of exchanges.

Everyone on the veterinary team plays a vital communication role. It takes a village to run a veterinary practice, care for people and their animals, and establish a functional practice team culture. Every conversation with clients and between colleagues impacts outcomes for the veterinary practice, and the resulting social dynamic affects veterinary practice team members, the clients served, and the patients cared for. Communication makes or breaks practice financial metrics, teamwork and morale, client satisfaction and adherence, and patient health. The return on developing veterinary team communication competence is multifold and an investment in patient care, client service, and team coordination. It literally pays dividends to invest in communication skills.

Equip Your Communication Toolbox

This book highlights 20 communication skills with proven success in navigating diverse clinical scenarios (Sidebar 1.1) (Appendix A). Taking a skills-based approach means we do not need a specific strategy for each routine or difficult conversation. Instead, we carry our toolbox to each scenario and pick the appropriate tools to accomplish the task. As a result, we are ready, agile, and adaptable to meet all day to day communication circumstances that present in veterinary practice.

Sidebar 1.1 Skills in the Communication Toolbox

Preparation
Introduction
Agenda-setting
Open-ended inquiry
Closed-ended inquiry
Pause
Minimal encouragers
Reflective listening
Nonverbal behaviors
Empathy
Partnership
Asking permission
Logical sequence
Signpost
Internal summary
Easily understood language
Chunk-and-check
End summary
Contracts for next steps
Final check

We rely on our communication toolbox to guide most routine client interactions, from preventive care topics, such as vaccinations, weight management, and dental hygiene, to complex end-of-life conversations, medical errors, and financial discussions. Equally important, bring our tools to collegial conversations; use them when interviewing potential employees, hosting team meetings, and conducting performance reviews. These skills are indispensable and an important part of every veterinary professional's development. Although all communication skills are highly pertinent and critical for success (Adams and Kurtz 2017; Silverman et al. 2013), effective communication requires a lifetime of mastery. So, as a starting point, we chose 20 foundational communication skills to stock the toolbox: once acquired, expand upon them.

Practice, Practice, Practice

Just like learning any clinical skill, such as navigating new practice management software, performing a surgical procedure, or interpreting radiographs, communication skill-building takes practice and time. We obtain the baseline knowledge through reading, attending a lecture, or completing an online module. Where the rubber meets the road is testing our competency in everyday practice. Once we get the underlying principles and concepts under our belt, the best way to learn communication skills is to "just do it." This allows us to apply our understanding of effective communication and form good habits through practice and experience.

The learning ladder (Figure 1.1) depicts four stages of learning new communication skills, from raising awareness to reaching mastery (DePhillips et al. 1960, Wackman et al. 1976). We do not know what we do not know. The first step is obtaining knowledge to raise awareness, answering for ourselves such questions as "What is the communication skill?", "What does it sound like?", and "When, why, and how might I use it?"

Awareness (we know what we do not know) is followed by a period of awkwardness as we put the new skill into practice. This stage is messy, feels inept, and demands courage, patience, perseverance, and a big, heaping dose of self-acceptance until we are consciously skilled. Like learning anything new, communicating differently feels strange and sounds unnatural; the words do not always come out right at first. This necessitates a shift in mindset away from expecting perfection to embracing the awkward.

With more feedback, practice, and reflection, communication skills fall into place. Initially, using a communication skill requires a great deal of mental effort, concentration, and purposeful intent, like when we learn to ride a horse, pedal a bike, drive a car, or ski. Eventually, proficiency is achieved, competence becomes unconsciously integrated, and the skills are automatic and habitual.

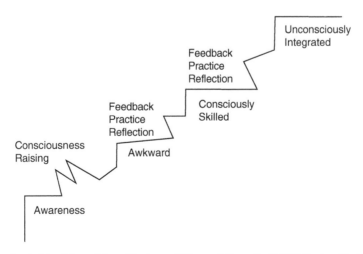

Figure 1.1 Learning ladder. Adapted from Wackman, Miller, and Nunnally, (1976) *Student Workbook: Increasing Awareness and Communication Skills*-with permission from Interpersonal Communication Programs, LLC, Evergreen, CO. USA.

This learning process demands being forgiving of ourselves, letting go, and being all right with not getting it right the first time around. Dr. Tracy Jensen, a primary-care veterinarian, consultant, and communication coach at Colorado State University College of Veterinary Medicine and Biomedical Sciences, says, "If you are not falling, you are not skiing hard enough." If we are not stretching ourselves outside our comfort zone, we are not learning. So, lean into the challenge of learning these communication skills and welcome the initial clumsiness that is often on the path to competence.

Appreciate Communication is An Art and a Science

Communication is about establishing trust **and** achieving outcomes. The field of medical communication was founded in 1968 (Korsch et al. 1968) and veterinary communication in 1988 (Antelyes 1988), and research touting the benefits of effective communication in healthcare is robust and persuasive. Thousands of studies in medical communication, including randomized clinical trials (Silverman et al. 2013), and hundreds of studies in veterinary communication (Adams and Kurtz 2017) inform best practices. The communication toolbox provided in this book is fortified by a database of literature and evidence-based recommendations.

You might recall a role model sharing, "It's not what you say, it's how you say it"; truthfully, it is both. Communication content is **what** we say (i.e. the science), and it comprises the biomedical background and experience required for effective information-gathering and client education. The communication process is **how** we say it (i.e. the art), or how we come across when we ask questions, provide explanations, or support decisions. For the message (the content) to be received, it comes down to our delivery (the process), which requires paying close attention to the communication skills used.

The science of communication entails using the skills with purpose and intention. Many of us did not receive formal training in communication skills and were schooled painfully by trial and error. With knowledge of communication skills and their impact on clinical outcomes – like choosing instruments from a surgical pack – we select the best communication tool or tools at the appropriate time to target and achieve our sought-after outcomes.

The art of communication reflects our ability to apply the skills adeptly not only in straightforward interactions but also in nuanced, complex, challenging, and high-stakes situations with diverse individuals. One size does not fit all. An indication of communication mastery is the ability to be fully present in the moment, quickly assess the scenario, and implement our communication skills accordingly. A high level of proficiency is also demonstrated in keen self-awareness, noticing when an interaction goes off the rails, and the ability to make a prompt repair and recovery.

Build, Maintain, and Sustain Relationships

A common retort we receive during communication workshops is "I'm not a counselor." So, let's get this straight up front: we are not asking, expecting, or training you to be or become a therapist, as you, a veterinary professional, are not equipped or licensed to provide psychological counseling. However, we are strong proponents of building relationships and supporting clients and colleagues for success in veterinary practice. Dr. Matthew Johnston, an avian, exotic, and zoo veterinarian and communication coach at Colorado State University College of Veterinary Medicine and Biomedical Sciences, says, "If you use effective communication, you won't need to be a counselor."

Veterinary medicine was established in the eighteenth century with a focus on animal healthcare. With the cultural shift in our views and uses of animals and the transformation of the human-animal bond, it is now a "people profession." Veterinary medicine serves animals **and** the people who care for them. The daily challenge in a busy practice is balancing attending to tasks and relationships. It entails embracing both roles – as animal healthcare expert as well as partners to our clients and colleagues.

The desire to help our patients using the scientific mind leads us naturally down a path of "find it, fix it." There's a downside, however, to this apparent efficiency. We miss things. Make assumptions. Make a mess of an interaction, even misdiagnose. When drilling clients, like a detective interrogating their suspect, we drive our agenda forward and neglect to invite client contributions. With insufficient information-gathering and understanding, we prescribe treatments that a client cannot administer, afford, or get on board with. In our rush to finish the appointment on time, we unintentionally run over the animal's advocate. The result is a time-consuming snarl to untangle, and efficiency goes out the door.

Retired emergency veterinarian and Colorado State University College of Veterinary Medicine and Biomedical Sciences communication instructor, Dr. Sam Romano says, "Go slow to go fast." This means listening more, being curious, and acknowledging client perspectives, backgrounds, and experiences. Doing so pays off with efficiencies later in the interaction. We are often fearful of opening a can of worms and not knowing what to do with them, or how to respond to, what is shared. And we are always afraid of running behind. It seems paradoxical, but slowing down now with a client and showing patience and the courage to listen reaps rewards and time savings in the end. Take the time to be present. Empathize and collaborate to build trust, buy-in, and commitment – these are the critical ingredients for client adherence, satisfaction, and long-term client retention.

Enhance Clinical Outcomes

Communication impacts clinical outcomes at every level – for the veterinary practice; our colleagues, clients, and patients; and, importantly, ourselves (Sidebar 1.2). From generating a sustainable client base to retaining talented team members to ensuring that our patients receive the care they need, it all comes down to communication. Be purposeful and intentional, focusing on communicating, to achieve desired outcomes with colleagues, clients, and patients.

Sidebar 1.2 Clinical Outcomes of Effective Communication

Veterinary Practice

Enhance efficiency
Reduce malpractice claims
Improve practice performance

Veterinary Team

Foster satisfaction

Clients

Increase recall and understanding
Promote adherence
Cultivate satisfaction

Patients

Boost health

For the Veterinary Practice

Enhance Efficiency

Time management is one of the greatest day to day challenges in veterinary practice. A common misperception is that partner-oriented appointments take longer. Building relationships is the ticket to getting down to business. Invite clients to share their thoughts, feelings, and ideas; and listen closely, as clients who feel heard are ready to problem-solve, tackle decision-making, and accept a plan.

To better manage appointment time, elicit the client's agenda up front to meet their expectations and mindfully structure the appointment (Dysart et al. 2011). If unable to address all the client's concerns, prioritize – and seek alternative approaches, such as a drop-off or a recheck visit. Pace with the client during diagnostic and treatment planning to identify concerns and address obstacles, detours, or roadblocks in the moment. Ask "What else?" throughout the appointment to avoid an "Oh, by the way" moment at the end (Dysart et al. 2011).

Reduce Malpractice Claims

A strong foundation of trust and a resilient client relationship provide a cushion when things go wrong. Set a tone of collaboration upfront, make authentic connections with clients, and ask them about themselves. Listen to their stories and how they share observations on the animals with whom they live and believe in the client's expertise. Build rapport to enhance information-gathering and subsequent diagnostic accuracy to minimize medical errors (Dinsmore and McConnell 1992). A trusting relationship carries the partnership through good times and bad. Clients know that we as veterinary professionals are imperfect human beings. When we let clients see our goodwill, compassion, and underlying intention to keep their best interests in mind, regardless of outcome, they will be more understanding and forgiving.

Improve Practice Performance

Communication that builds client and collegial relationships is the bread and butter of a successful veterinary practice. Connect with clients to enhance efficiency (Dysart et al. 2011), promote client adherence (Kanji et al. 2012) and satisfaction, and improve patient health – all of which directly affect the bottom line. Revenue is generated when patients receive the healthcare they need and clients the quality service they expect. The result is meeting the metrics of practice success, including average client transactions, return client visits, client referrals, a healthy client base, and positive client reviews, while attending to patient care. A base of loyal clients is critical to practice financial performance, and so is a core team of content and dedicated employees. Equally important is the recruitment and retention of talented team members, resulting from appreciation and recognition, opportunities for professional development, and a healthy workplace culture (Moore et al. 2014; Pizzolon et al. 2019).

For the Veterinary Team

Foster Satisfaction

Professional wellness is a major factor in the health, well-being, and longevity of veterinary professionals (Nett et al. 2015). The ability to successfully navigate difficult discussions is related to veterinarian and client well-being. When unsuccessful, veterinarians experience a reduced sense of well-being and job satisfaction, increased emotional strain, and detrimental client impact. For example, facilitating the euthanasia decision-making conversation was found to be more challenging than performing the euthanasia procedure (Matte et al. 2019).

One of the protective factors against compassion fatigue is the fulfillment derived from interactions with teammates and clients (Cake et al. 2015). Client and team interactions are a source of professional fulfillment (Moore et al. 2014; Pizzolon et al. 2019; Shaw et al. 2012) and reduce stress and burnout (Moore et al. 2014, 2015). Improving teamwork reduces medical errors, a major stressor for veterinary professionals (Cummings et al. 2022). Enjoying work with our clients and colleagues boosts team morale and makes the veterinary practice a fun, engaging, and empowering place to work.

For Clients

Increase Recall and Understanding
It is often challenging for clients to comprehend all the details, jargon, and descriptions related to their animal's disease, diagnostic tests, or treatment plan. Before launching into one of our well-honed spiels, in the name of client education, stop and assess what the client knows already, to tailor information directly to them. Gauge the depth of their knowledge, and identify their communication preferences to provide the level of detail they desire and present information in a way that makes sense to them. To enhance client understanding, translate foreign medical terminology and speak in layman's terms. Take complex medical concepts and break them into bite-sized pieces. Invite clients to ask questions throughout the appointment, check in frequently, and ask them to repeat back what they are hearing to increase their recall and understanding (Stoewen et al. 2014a).

Promote Adherence
Clients are more likely to accept recommendations from a professional with whom they have a trusting relationship. Trust-building starts with identifying our clients' concerns, goals, expectations, and priorities up front so we meet their needs (Dysart et al. 2011). To further develop the relationship, provide empathy, care, and compassion and offer partnership throughout the visit. Elicit client's perspective to identify their caregiving strengths and potential challenges that need to be overcome. Then tailor a plan that fits the client and patient. Involve the client at every step, as an actively engaged client is more likely to adhere to recommendations (Kanji et al. 2012).

Cultivate Satisfaction
In many regions, clients have choices when seeking veterinary care for their animals. Interestingly, their decisions are not based on our grades in veterinary school, diagnostic brilliance, or surgical ability, but rather on their perception of how much the veterinary team cares (Brown and Silverman 1999). As Theodore Roosevelt said, "People don't care how much you know, until they know how much you care." It is the one-on-one relationship that often brings a client back, so invest in clients and their pets to foster long-term relationships and retention. How much we care comes through in the way we interact with the animal, introduce ourselves, listen to the client's concerns, provide support, and demonstrate interest in, relate to, and connect with the client (Coe et al. 2008; Stoewen et al. 2014b).

For Patients

Boost Health

Clients are our conduit for applying our medical knowledge and delivering the medical care that pets need. As veterinary professionals, we need to build trust and engage clients as partners in their pet's healthcare. We rely on the client to share key data to make an accurate diagnosis, to give permission for diagnostic and treatment options, and to provide at-home nursing care for the pet.

Foster Veterinary Team Culture

Day to day interactions between veterinary colleagues, ranging from social chit-chat to critical life-saving instructions, are the foundation of team communication. Highly functional team conversations build a practice environment of trust and respect. And a trusting practice culture creates positive work processes, promotes colleague recruitment and retention, and fosters team engagement, morale, and satisfaction.

Team communication makes the difference between a healthy practice environment and a dysfunctional one; enjoying work or dreading it; flourishing in an open and trusting atmosphere or wilting from gossip, back-stabbing, competitive one-upmanship, and tip-toeing around each other; and taking initiative or being fearful of making a mistake (Moore et al. 2015). It's not surprising then that a colleague's decision to quit or dedicate their life's work to our clinical practice comes down to the quality of the practice culture. Highly functional teams nurture fulfillment, contentment, and meaning, which preserve a long career in veterinary medicine (Moore et al. 2014; Pizzolon et al. 2019).

Coordinate Relationships

Veterinary teams with high relational coordination possess common goals, share knowledge, and demonstrate mutual respect (Gittell 2003). With shared goals, team members envision common targets and outcomes and value working together to achieve them. With shared knowledge, colleagues not only appreciate each other's roles and empathize with each other's challenges but also are competently cross-trained to step in for each other when needed. The emphasis on interdependence engenders mutual respect, as individuals recognize, grasp, and appreciate the contributions of others.

Achieving relational coordination within a veterinary team requires frequent, timely, accurate, and problem-solving communication (Gittell 2003). The team "spider web" (Figure 1.2) depicts the communication pattern of relational coordination. When team members communicate and check in regularly with their colleagues, they manifest their best selves within their roles and responsibilities and those of their colleagues. On the other hand, the spider web portrays how easy it is to unintentionally drop information between hand-offs, forget to pass a message on, or exclude someone from a conversation.

Establishing relational coordination means balancing team communication that nurtures relationships (i.e. builds a cohesive team) while completing tasks (i.e. gets the work done). This is a difficult juggling act in a hectic environment. Often the day to day demands of a fast-paced veterinary practice favor task-oriented communication over relational, placing team engagement at risk.

The challenge is looking at each individual interaction and how it contributes to team building, function, and effectiveness. This focus pays off in dividends, including career satisfaction and fulfillment (Moore et al. 2014; Pizzolon et al. 2019), improved task efficiency (Gittell 2009), healthier

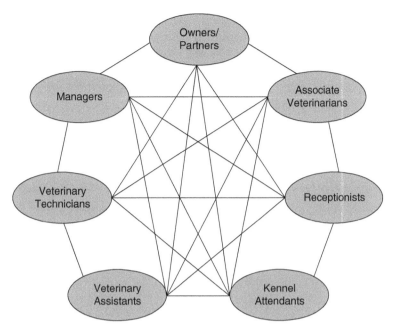

Figure 1.2 Relational coordination. Adapted from Gittell (2009) with permission.

patients (Gittell 2009), decreased burnout and cynicism (Moore et al. 2014), and reduced costs of care (Gittell 2009). The bottom line is creating a supportive, engaging, creative, and productive workplace that fosters fun, enjoyment, and fulfillment for all.

Make Time to Communicate

Over the years, one of the most common rebuttals we hear in teaching communication to veterinary students and professionals is "I don't have time for this." It is not the quantity of time spent with clients that is ultimately of greatest importance; it is the quality of the time together. For both the client and the veterinary professional, being distracted and hurried detracts from the experience, while being present and engaged nourishes the interaction. Client adherence is reduced when veterinary professionals are perceived as rushed (Kanji et al. 2012).

Reflect upon the "quantity versus quality" proposition, and assess your practice culture – is it defined by high-volume quantity or high-touch quality of appointments? The differentiator tends to be appointment length – 10- to 15-minutes in high-volume clinics compared to 20- to 30-minute appointments in high-touch clinics. A mixed model is flexible scheduling, such as 15-minutes for a recheck examination, 30-minutes for a wellness appointment, 45-minutes for a sick-pet appointment, and 1-hour for a new puppy or geriatric visit.

Especially in fast-paced, high-volume practices, prudent implementation of top-notch communication skills improves client service and patient care when there is not a minute to spare. Effective communication is possible during even the shortest appointments; doing so is challenging and requires a highly skilled and attentive communicator. The key is providing an opportunity for clients to share and feel heard. These relationship-centered appointments can be more efficient than traditional biomedically oriented appointments (Shaw et al. 2006).

The aim of this book is to create highly skilled and attentive communicators. We hope to compel you to invest in developing your communication skills and equip you with a strong communication toolbox to build relationships with clients and colleagues. Then use the communication skills with purpose and intention to achieve clinical outcomes for the practice, your colleagues, clients, patients, and, importantly, yourself. We wish for each of your interactions to foster a long-lasting, fulfilling, and meaningful career in veterinary medicine.

Answer Key

1. Effective communication can be learned through practice, feedback, and coaching. [True]
2. Effective communication is critical to achieving significant outcomes for the veterinary practice; with colleagues, clients, and patients; and self. [True]
3. Effective communication is integral to maintaining and sustaining a healthy practice culture and interprofessional relationships. [True]
4. Effective communication takes more time. [False]

References

Adams, C.A. and Kurtz, S.M. (2017). *Skills for Communicating in Veterinary Medicine*. Parsippany, NJ: Dewpoint Publishing.

Antelyes, J. (1988). Talking to clients. *J. Am. Vet. Med. Assoc.* 193 (12): 1502–1504.

Brown, J.P. and Silverman, J.D. (1999). The current and future market for veterinarians and veterinary medical services in the United States. *J. Am. Vet. Med. Assoc.* 215 (2): 161–183.

Cake, M.A., Bell, M.A., Bickley, N., and Bartram, D.A. (2015). The life of meaning: a model of positive contributions to well-being from veterinary work. *J. Vet. Med. Educ.* 42 (3): 184–193. https://doi.org/10.3138/jvme.1014-097R1.

Coe, J.B., Adams, C.L., and Bonnett, B.N. (2008). A focus group study of veterinarians' and pet owners' perceptions of veterinarian-client communication in companion animal practice. *J. Am. Vet. Med. Assoc.* 233 (7): 1072–1080. https://doi.org/10.2460/javma.233.7.1072.

Cummings, C.O., Krucik, D.D.R., Carroll, J.P., and Eisenbarth, J.M. (2022). Improving within-team communication to reduce the risk of medical errors. *J. Am. Vet. Med. Assoc.* 260 (6): 600–602. https://doi.org/10.2460/javma.21.09.0407.

DePhillips, F.A., Berliner W.M., and Cribbin, J.J. (1960). Management of Training Programs. Richard D. Erwin.

Dinsmore, J. and McConnell, D. (1992). Communication to avoid malpractice claims. *J. Am. Vet. Med. Assoc.* 201 (3): 283–287.

Dysart, M.A., Coe, J.B., and Adams, C.L. (2011). Analysis of solicitation of client concerns in companion animal practice. *J. Am. Vet. Med. Assoc.* 238 (12): 1609–1615. https://doi.org/10.2460/javma.238.12.1609.

Gittell, J.H. (2003). *The Southwest Airlines Way: Using the Power of Relationships to Achieve High Performance*. New York, NY: McGraw-Hill.

Gittell, J.H. (2009). *High Performance Healthcare: Using the Power of Relationships to Achieve Quality, Efficiency and Resilience*. New York, NY: McGraw-Hill.

Kanji, N., Coe, J.B., Adams, C.L., and Shaw, J.R. (2012). Effect of veterinarian-client-patient interactions on client adherence to dentistry and surgery recommendations in companion animal practice. *J. Am. Vet. Med. Assoc.* 240 (4): 427–436. https://doi.org/10.2460/javma.240.4.427.

Korsch, B.M., Gozzi, E.K., and Francis, V. (1968). Gaps in doctor-patient communication: doctor-patient interaction and patient satisfaction. *Pediatrics* 42 (5): 855–871.

Matte, A.R., Khosa, D.K., Coe, J.B., and Meehan, M.P. (2019). Impacts of the process and decision-making around companion animal euthanasia on veterinary well-being. *Vet. Rec.* 185 (15): 1–6. https://doi.org/10.1136/vr.105540.

Moore, I.C., Coe, J.B., Adams, C.L. et al. (2014). The role of veterinary team effectiveness in job satisfaction and burnout in companion animal clinics. *J. Am. Vet. Med. Assoc.* 245 (5): 513–524. https://doi.org/10.2460/javma.245.5.513.

Moore, I.C., Coe, J.B., Adams, C.L. et al. (2015). Exploring the impact of toxic attitudes and toxic environment on the veterinary healthcare team. *Front. Vet. Sci.* 2: 78. https://doi.org/10.3389/fvets.2015.00078.

Nett, R.J., Witte, T.K., Holzebauer, S.M. et al. (2015). Risk factors for suicide, attitudes toward mental illness, and practice-related stressors among US veterinarians. *J. Am. Vet. Med. Assoc.* 247 (8): 945–955. https://doi.org/10.2460/javma.247.8.945.

Pizzolon, C., Coe, J.B., and Shaw, J.R. (2019). The role of team effectiveness and personal empathy in veterinary personnel's professional quality of life and job satisfaction in companion animal practice. *J. Am. Vet. Med. Assoc.* 254 (10): 1204–1217. https://doi.org/10.2460/javma.254.10.1204.

Shaw, J.R., Bonnett, B.N., Adams, C.L., and Roter, D.L. (2006). Veterinarian-client-patient communication patterns used during clinical appointments in companion animal practice. *J. Am. Vet. Med. Assoc.* 228 (5): 714–721. https://doi.org/10.2460/javma.240.7.832.

Shaw, J.R., Adams, C.L., Bonnett, B.N. et al. (2012). Veterinarian satisfaction with veterinary visits. *J. Am. Vet. Med. Assoc.* 240 (7): 832–841. https://doi.org/10.2460/javma.228.5.714.

Silverman, J., Kurtz, S., and Draper, J. (2013). *Skills for Communicating with Patients*. London, England: CRC Press.

Stoewen, D.L., Coe, J.B., MacMartin, C. et al. (2014a). Qualitative study of the information expectations of clients assessing oncology care at a tertiary referral center for dogs with life-limiting cancer. *J. Am. Vet. Med. Assoc.* 245 (7): 773–783. https://doi.org/10.2460/javma.245.7.785.

Stoewen, D.L., Coe, J.B., MacMartin, C. et al. (2014b). Qualitative study of the communication expectations of clients assessing oncology care at a tertiary referral center for dogs with life-limiting cancer. *J. Am. Vet. Med. Assoc.* 245 (7): 785–795. https://doi.org/10.2460/javma.245.7.773.

Wackman, D.B., Miller, S., and Nunnally, E.W. (1976). *Student Workbook: Increasing Awareness and Communication Skills*. Interpersonal Communication Programs, LLC, Evergreen, CO. USA.

2

Communication Styles

Abstract

This chapter acknowledges that a paradigm shift is underway in the veterinary profession's relationship with clients. Today, more than ever, clients expect excellent customer service. Clients share strong bonds with their pets, conduct research on the internet, and speak out in reviews if their needs are not met. Clients are moving away from the previous paternalistic relationship and toward a collaborative partnership with their veterinary care provider. Many clients are no longer content with passivity and prefer to take an active role in the decision-making process and their animal's healthcare. The same is true in the workplace: veterinary colleagues want to be valued for their unique contribution, be engaged in their roles and responsibilities, and play an integral part on a high-performing team. In this chapter, we introduce four communication styles, with appropriate times and places to be used when interacting with clients and colleagues.

SELF-ASSESSMENT QUESTIONS

1. What is my preferred communication style: being an expert (i.e. taking the lead) or a partner (i.e. sharing the floor)? How does my style differ during client versus colleague interactions?
2. Think of a client or colleague. How do I determine their preferred communication style (i.e. expert versus partner)? What cues can I observe?
3. How do I align my communication style with that of my client or colleague, and what is the resulting impact on our interaction?

Introduction

A paradigm shift is underway with respect to the veterinary profession's relationship with clients. Today, more than ever, clients expect excellent customer service. Clients share strong bonds with their pets, conduct research on the internet, and speak out in reviews if their needs are not met. Clients are moving away from the previous paternalistic relationship style and toward a collaborative partnership with veterinary care providers (Coe et al. 2008; Shaw et al. 2006; Nogueira Borden et al. 2010; Janke et al. 2021).

Many clients are no longer content with passivity and prefer to take an active role in the decision-making process and their animal's healthcare (Coe et al. 2008; Janke et al. 2021). The same is true in the workplace; veterinary colleagues want to be valued for their unique contributions, be engaged in their roles and responsibilities, and play an integral part on a high-performing team (Moore et al. 2014, 2015; Pizzolon et al. 2019). Therefore, alignment of communication styles is paramount to achieving clinical outcomes for the veterinary practice, team, clients, patients, and ourselves (Sidebar 2.1).

Sidebar 2.1   Improved Clinical Outcomes of Aligning Communication Styles

Increase accuracy
Enhance efficiency
Foster client recall and understanding
Promote client satisfaction
Achieve client adherence
Improve patient health
Enhance veterinary professional satisfaction

Communication styles are the first topic of this book because they influence how to use the individual communication skills that follow in subsequent chapters. These styles reflect personality traits and leadership approaches, which are driven by underlying temperament and character. As a result, we possess a natural communication style that feels most comfortable to us, as well as a default style we lean on when stressed.

Despite possessing a preferred communication style, we flex in the moment beyond our comfort zone to use contrasting approaches as needed. Self-awareness, quick assessments, a strong communication toolbox, and adaptability are keys to success. In knowing our style and gauging that of others, we are poised to adapt to successfully engaging with clients and colleagues.

In this chapter, we introduce four communication styles, with appropriate times and paces – ideal situations or use – for interacting with clients and colleagues (Sidebar 2.2). We define each communication style, discuss its advantages and disadvantages, and provide scenarios for use. First we illustrate the communication styles in the context of a veterinary professional-client interaction in the Pearsons' and Titus's recheck visit with Gabe, the veterinary technician; then we apply them to a collegial interaction in a couple of meetings between Marta, the client service supervisor, and Theresa, the practice owner to resolve ongoing concerns about patient congestion at the front desk.

Sidebar 2.2   Communication Styles

Expert-in-charge
Expert-guide
Partner
Facilitator

Set the Scene

Client Scenario: The Pearsons present with Titus, a Staffordshire terrier, to recheck his right eye. Titus presented five days ago with swelling, redness, and third-eyelid protrusion in his eye. While Gabe, the veterinary technician, focuses on his priorities, the Pearsons' frustration mounts, as they are seeking a collaborative approach to care for Titus.

Team Scenario: Marta, the client service supervisor, is concerned about client and patient congestion at the front desk. Clients are angry about being placed on hold while on the phone and waiting far too long to check in or out. Marta is worried about patient safety with animals so close to each other in the queue at the front desk. The entire client service team is flustered from juggling too many tasks at once. So, Marta, who likes to brainstorm options, requests a meeting with Theresa, the authoritative, no-nonsense practice owner.

Stepping into Gabe's and Marta's shoes, self-reflect on the following:

1. How would I diffuse the Pearsons' frustration and meet them as a partner?
2. How might I approach "get-down-to-business" Theresa with my concerns?

Adapt Communication Styles to Clients

One Shoe Does Not Fit All

The four communication styles are laid out on the graph in Figure 2.1. Let's walk through the communication styles, from expert-in-charge to facilitator. A veterinary professional's placement

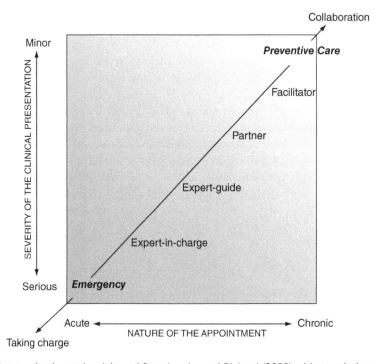

Figure 2.1 Communication styles. Adapted from Lussier and Richard (2008) with permission.

on the graph is based on who is doing the most talking, the nature of the appointment, and the severity of the medical problem (Lussier and Richard 2008).

Who Is Doing the Talking?

In Figure 2.1, the four communication styles are plotted along a gradient. In the lower-left quadrant, the veterinary professional dominates the conversation, and there is low client participation. The expert-in-charge or expert-guide do most of the talking and drive their agenda. In the upper-right quadrant, there is minimal veterinary professional conversation and high client participation; here, partners or facilitators, share the dialogue and co-create the agenda with their client.

Role of Appointment Type and Severity of the Medical Problem

Although many factors sway the choice of communication style for each situation, Lussier and Richard (2008) focus on two aspects: the nature of the appointment (i.e. acute or chronic) and the severity of the clinical presentation (i.e. serious or minor). In veterinary medicine, appointment type – a preventive care exam or a consultation for a health-related problem – was found to influence veterinarians' communication style (Shaw et al. 2008).

When caring for a pet during an acute emergency, such as a hit-by-car, gastric-dilatation and volvulus, or pericardial effusion, the veterinary team initially directs the conversation, taking a strong leadership role as expert-in-charge (i.e. lower-left quadrant). The focus is on stabilizing the patient. The goal is to provide clients with enough information to make a timely, informed decision. Once the animal is out of danger, a shift in communication style occurs to allow for collaborative decision-making to address treatment of the underlying injuries or disease.

In contrast, speaking with a client whose pet has a less urgent, chronic disease – diabetes mellitus, osteoarthritis, or hyperthyroidism – or needs preventive care calls for a facilitative approach (i.e. upper-right quadrant). In this scenario, the client serves as an expert because of their knowledge of and copious experience caring for the pet. The veterinary professional provides guidance, monitors progress, and adjusts the treatment plan to optimize the pet's quality of life.

Communication styles are dynamic, and we flex within and between appointments. Even though we prefer a particular communication style, we adapt to the clinical scenario, the patient, and the client in front of us. To do so, we need to develop a full repertoire of communication styles, as truly, **one shoe does not fit all** clients, patients, or colleagues.

Communication Styles

Expert

In this context, the term "expert" refers to a communication style, which is independent of education level, acquired knowledge, or specialty. All veterinary team members possess expertise; it is how we communicate that to our clients and colleagues that is important. Even more crucial is how our clients and colleagues prefer to receive information.

Experts (i.e. expert-in-charge and expert-guide roles) tend to dominate the agenda for the appointment, assume the client's values are the same as theirs, and take on the role of a guardian for the patient (Roter et al. 2000 and Shaw et al. 2006). Because experts take the lead, clients play a more passive role, and the veterinary professional often prioritizes the needs of the pet over those of the client. Traditionally, the expert role is the most common approach to medical and veterinary visits (Shaw et al. 2006). Other terminology related to the expert role is "biomedical communication" (Shaw et al. 2006) or "veterinarian-centered communication or care."

Expert communication is depicted by a **shot-put** for its unilateral delivery of information that is large in mass and scale (Barbour 2000; Kurtz et al. 2005). The intent is to efficiently complete a task, with the focus on the outcome, less so on the process of getting there. Therefore, the expert approach offers clear, direct, quick communication that exudes and instills confidence. An expert takes decisive, potentially life-saving action and moves an agenda forward (Sidebar 2.3).

Sidebar 2.3   Expert Communication Style

Advantages

Provides education
Delivers timely care
Addresses emergencies

Disadvantages

Feels overwhelming
Contributes to misalignment
Coerces decisions
Rushes decision-making
Risks regrets
Potentiates blame

The challenge is that the sender often assumes the client received, processed, and agreed with the delivered message. So, in the expert atmosphere, it is critical to acknowledge that clients may be reluctant to speak up if they think differently. Clients may feel steamrolled or pressured to do as recommended and may resent or regret the chosen plan later. Experts may not achieve buy-in to their plan or their desired outcomes.

Partner

In this book, we refer to partnering in two different ways. In this chapter, we present the partner communication style that seeks to establish a collaborative veterinary professional-client or collegial relationship. Then, in Chapter 5, we introduce the use of partnership language (i.e. *we, us, let's, together*) to express our desire to "work with" the client or colleague as a team. Such partnership statements pave the way to establishing strong, trusting, mutual relationships.

Partners (i.e. partner and facilitator roles) strive for a balance of power and mutuality between veterinary professional and client (Roter et al. 2000 and Shaw et al. 2006). Being a service professional means melding our agenda with that of the client to meet, if not exceed, client expectations. Partners advocate simultaneously for client and patient needs alongside their recommendations and strive to reach common ground. Related terminology includes "biolifestyle-social communication" (Shaw et al. 2006) and "relationship-" or "client-centered communication or care."

Partner interactions are characterized by negotiation and the creation of a joint venture. Collaboration is a necessary and critical ingredient to achieve desirable outcomes. To do so, partners incorporate their client's perspective, values, and beliefs into all phases of the consultation: agenda-setting, information-gathering, diagnostic and treatment planning, and decision-making. Although partners are client-centered, they voice their concerns, provide medical information, state professional opinions, and insert their agenda into the conversation. However, using the partnership model, they are cognizant of when and how they do so and examine the potential consequences.

Partner communication is symbolized by a **Frisbee**, emphasizing the reciprocal exchange of information and adjusting messages to stay on target (Barbour 2000; Kurtz et al. 2005). The intent is on the journey – how we will get to the outcome – rather than the destination. Partners assess how the client perceives, processes, and understands the message before going on. The strengths of partnership are dialoguing, eliciting feedback, and checking to ensure that both parties are moving forward together (Sidebar 2.4).

Sidebar 2.4 Partner Communication Style

Advantages

Enhances relationships
Builds trust
Engages in discussion
Improves understanding and recall
Promotes adherence
Fosters client satisfaction
Enriches veterinarian satisfaction

Disadvantages

Takes time up front
Lacks decisive direction
Demands resources
Delays decision-making

The challenge is that it may take longer, and we may not have the required time to achieve the desired result. Also, not every client wants to collaborate; some individuals expect a direct answer or clear guidance. If structure, organization, and facilitation are lacking, it is difficult to maintain momentum and direction using a partner-based approach, halting progress.

Align Styles to Achieve Outcomes

To recap, the challenge of the expert communication style is that it is unilateral. Intuitively, the expert approach seems quick and efficient; however, it may not be so. When "experts" force agendas or plans on their clients, it is difficult to reach agreement, move forward, and achieve full client buy-in. To overcome these roadblocks, "experts" often need to step back and revisit eliciting the client's perspective, commitments, and beliefs, taking more time during the front end of the appointment.

Partner-based communication often takes more time up front during opening-the-interaction and information-gathering due to eliciting contributions from others and building an atmosphere of trust. But after the foundation is laid, time is made up, and progress is quick during diagnostic and treatment planning and closing-the-interaction. Contrary to common perception, the net effect is that partnership-oriented appointments take less time (Research Spotlight 2.1). Not only that, but the path forward is smoother and often more fulfilling, from working with long-term, devoted, and loyal clients.

> **Research Spotlight 2.1**
>
> **Biomedical Appointments Take Longer**
>
> In a quantitative analysis of primary care appointments, relationship-centered appointments (i.e. partner-based) took significantly less time (mean $= 10.43$ minutes) than biomedical appointments (i.e. expert-based, mean $= 11.98$ minutes, $p = 0.02$) (Shaw et al. 2006). Although a 1.55-minute difference in means between communication styles seems slight, it adds up quickly with multiple appointments in a day. Take time up front in the appointment to gather the client's agenda and their perspective, and to build a trusting relationship.

Meet as Experts

Our clients are experts in understanding their pets and themselves. They know the animal's lifestyle, the household environment, and possess extensive background information. In addition, clients are cognizant of their schedules, resource limitations, and ideas, beliefs, and values. Clients represent half the equation, and without their input, we may find ourselves battling client adherence issues, a lack of understanding, or poor client satisfaction. Discussing details such as financial resources, who is the pet's primary caregiver, how easy or difficult it will be to implement a treatment plan, or recent life changes (e.g. birth or death, new job, recent move) allows you to tailor the treatment plan and promote client adherence.

A true partnership is a meeting of experts through honoring the "expert" in each – our expertise in animal healthcare and the client's expertise in their pet and their life circumstances. More satisfying outcomes result from bringing the two together into what may at first sound like a paradoxical relationship: a partnership of experts.

Embrace Diversity

Diversity in veterinary practice includes differences not only in the countries, regions, and cultures in which we work but also in individual clients, patients, disease presentations, appointment types, and schedules. This variety presents a gift and a challenge. The reward is that no one day is the same, and we embrace each scenario as it comes. The difficulty is seeing and meeting each client, clinical case, or patient where they are.

Multiple factors influence how we use communication styles. Table 2.1 depicts general trends for each factor; it is far from predictive of individual scenarios, nor are these aspects mutually exclusive, as many considerations may come into play simultaneously. Therefore, we assess each client and the clinical situation mindfully and carefully on a case-by-case basis to determine how to best align communication styles.

Be Flexible

Each communication style has its place in client interactions and plays an important and integral role in achieving goals. Positive outcomes are more likely to be achieved when styles are aligned, such as when both parties prefer a partner or an expert communication style (Sidebar 2.1). That's when the listed advantages of the communication styles prevail. Challenges are more likely to arise during discordant expert-partner interactions, when the outlined disadvantages of the communication styles predominate (Sidebars 2.3 and 2.4).

Table 2.1 Factors that may influence the use of communication styles.

Factor	Expert communication style	Partner communication style
Veterinary practice culture	Focus on the number of clients visiting the practice	Focus on the quality of client experience
Veterinary specialty	Emergency and critical care Surgery Cardiology Neurology	Primary care Internal medicine Dermatology Oncology
Veterinary professional or client demeanor, character, and personality	High task orientation – get it done	High relational orientation – build trust and rapport
Veterinarian gender (Research Spotlight 2.2)	Male	Female
Veterinary professional or client generation	Baby Boomer and Gen X	Gen Y and Z
Level of client veterinary expertise	Low knowledge and experience	High knowledge and experience
Number of appointments/day	20–25	10–15
Length of appointment	5–15 min	20–30 min
Type of appointment (Research Spotlight 2.3)	Emergency or health problem	Preventive care
Human–animal bond	Functional or utilitarian attachment	Strong companion attachment

---

Research Spotlight 2.2

Veterinarian Gender Influences Communication Style

In a quantitative analysis of primary care appointments, female-identifying veterinarians displayed a significantly greater relationship-centered communication (RCC) style (i.e. partner) compared with male-identifying veterinarians (RCC score equaled 0.98 for females and 0.79 for males) (Shaw et al. 2012). Male veterinarians were more likely to take on an expert approach and female veterinarians a partnership approach. These findings highlight that although we might tend toward a particular communication style, we may need to flex to the communication style of our client.

Research Spotlight 2.3

Appointment Type Influences Communication Style

Veterinarian communication styles differ significantly based on appointment type (Shaw et al. 2006). In 31% of preventive care visits and 85% of health problem visits, veterinarians used a biomedical communication pattern (i.e. expert). In 69% of preventive visits and 15% of health problem visits, veterinarians used a biolifestyle-social communication pattern (i.e. partner). Health problem visits tended to be more task-oriented, with veterinary professionals taking on the role of expert, while preventive care visits were more relational, with time spent building trust and collaborative partnerships. These findings emphasize the importance of taking time to build strong and mutual relationships in both preventive care and health problem visits.

We can imagine beyond the two-dimensional diagram that veterinary professionals spend their day rollerblading along the diagonal line in Figure 2.1. We switch communication styles to align with clients between and even within appointments (Research Spotlight 2.4). Being a "client relationship ninja" requires being present and flexible: observing what is happening, calibrating responses to each situation, and adjusting in the moment. It is our job to promote effective communication. So, this responsibility – to meet the communication style of the other – falls on the shoulders of the veterinary professional.

Research Spotlight 2.4

Veterinarians Use Both Communication Styles

In an evaluation of the communication patterns of 50 veterinarians, 46% used predominantly the biomedical communication pattern (i.e. expert), 38% used a mixed communication pattern (i.e. expert and partner), and 16% used primarily the biolifestyle-social communication pattern (i.e. partner) (Shaw et al. 2012). Based on this evidence, it is important for veterinary professionals to adapt their communication style to their appointments and the clients standing before them.

Responsiveness is key, as communication styles change within an interaction, between interactions with the same individual, and between appointments. For instance, in an emergency, the veterinary professional, client, and patient usually need an expert to assess the problem, stabilize the animal, and formulate an initial diagnostic and care plan. This ensures patient safety and prompt treatment in a life-threatening situation. After the patient is stabilized, the veterinary professional may transition to be a partner: sitting down, eliciting the client's agenda and perspective, explaining the presumptive diagnosis, and exploring a care plan for moving forward where both parties contribute and become invested.

Make a Recovery When Needed

As human beings, we will not always get things right: misjudgments will be made, conversations will take detours, and communication styles will not mesh. When tensions rise, when someone withdraws or checks out of the conversation, or when an individual dominates the conversation, it is normal to sense stress. Note what is happening, and take a mental step back and a deep breath to see the clues indicating that the interaction went awry.

The good news is that it is possible to make a recovery. There are almost always opportunities to reset: to start over, identify the preferred style of the other, and quickly adjust our communication style to meet theirs. When a discussion gets off to a wrong start: apologize, acknowledge what went wrong, and begin reparations. Most individuals are willing to forgive, forget, and start over.

Commonly Asked Questions Related to Client Communication Styles

Clients Want an Authoritative Expert. Isn't That Why They Come to See Me?

That is true; we are veterinary medical experts. Clients seek animal healthcare expertise, and we are well equipped to deliver. What differs is how clients prefer to be educated and their level of engagement. Some want someone to take charge and tell them what to do; they are eager and ready to be filled up with information like a vessel. And other clients want to be included in decision-making; they prefer to play an active role in the dynamic and participate in an exchange tailored to their individual needs, backgrounds, and special concerns for their pets. Our role is to assess and determine the client's preferences and align our communication style appropriately.

I Prefer to Form Partnerships with My Clients. Can't I Stick to That?

In many and perhaps most cases, yes. However, some clients display a "get down to business" attitude. They put experts at ease but stretch partner-based professionals outside of their comfort zones because they want direct, clear leadership – they may need a confident, "take charge" stance to trust the veterinary professional's judgment. Also, regardless of a client's style preference, we need to take charge during emergencies. These are opportunities to flex the expert communication style to meet the needs of our clients and patients.

Client Scenario

Set the Scene: The Pearsons present with Titus, a Staffordshire terrier, to recheck his right eye (previous swelling, redness, and third-eyelid protrusion). Gabe, the veterinary technician, gathers the initial history.

> **GABE:** *Hello, Mrs. Pearson, Mr. Pearson. I see you're here for a recheck on Titus's right eye. How's he been doing?*
>
> **MRS. PEARSON:** *After our last appointment, I called our breeder, and she thinks it is Horner's syndrome. We do not know what to think. How can we figure this out?*
>
> **GABE:** *How did Titus do with the eye ointment?*
>
> **MRS. PEARSON:** *I followed the instructions to a "T," and there's a little improvement.*
>
> **GABE:** *How is Titus doing other than his eye?*
>
> **MR. PEARSON BREAKS IN:** *Our neighbor, who also has a terrier, thought it could be a tooth abscess pushing on the eye. We are getting different opinions and don't know what to believe. We want to know how to get Titus better.*
>
> **GABE:** *How is Titus's appetite?*
>
> **MRS. PEARSON:** *You know, frankly, we were dismayed that the veterinarian just gave us some eye ointment and sent us on our way. Dr. O'Brien was not interested in our questions, thoughts, or concerns. She told us what to do, regardless of whether it worked for us.*
>
> **MR. PEARSON:** *We just want to know what is going on, work together to treat it, and prevent it from happening again!*

Before reading on, reflect on the following three questions:

1. Which communication style(s) are the Pearsons favoring?
2. Which communication style is Gabe using?
3. What is the likely outcome?

Recovery Client Scenario

Set the Scene: In the previous scenario, the Pearsons were favoring a partner style: someone to listen to their thoughts and work with them to resolve the problem. Gabe exhibited an expert communication style by sticking to his priorities and ignoring the Pearsons' concerns. Due to the misalignment, the Pearsons may leave the practice dissatisfied and seek veterinary care elsewhere or rely on other sources for guidance, such as their breeder and neighbor. Therefore, in recognizing this and to recover the scenario, Gabe adjusts by switching communication styles and improves the interaction and, hopefully, the Pearsons' trust.

GABE: *Let's back up a minute. Tell me more about your last appointment with us.*

MRS. PEARSON: *Like I said, the doctor just gave us some eye ointment.*

GABE: *How do you think Titus responded to the eye ointment?*

MRS. PEARSON: *His eye looks a little better, but we can still see his third eyelid.*

GABE: *What are you hoping for today?*

MR. PEARSON: *The veterinarian didn't educate us on what was going on, what the diagnosis was called, or what to expect. So, I called our breeder, and she thinks it is Horner's syndrome.*

GABE: *I will share with Dr. O'Brien that you want a clearer explanation.*

MR. PEARSON: *I think our neighbor is probably right – it's a tooth-root abscess. I want to know what Dr. O'Brien thinks is going on and for her to share her thoughts with us.*

GABE: *So, you want to be educated on the diagnosis. You are concerned it could be Horner's syndrome or a tooth-root abscess. What else can we do to regain your confidence?*

MR. PEARSON: *Once we have a diagnosis, we want to work with Dr. O'Brien on how to treat it and how to prevent it in the future.*

GABE: *We'll do our best to involve you in each step. What else can we do to take care of you and Titus today?*

MR. PEARSON: *That's pretty much it, thank you.*

GABE: *We'll figure this out together. I will share your concerns about getting a clear diagnosis and an explanation, and being involved in Titus's care plan with Dr. O'Brien.*

Before reading on, again, reflect on the following three questions:

1. Which communication style(s) are the Pearsons favoring?
2. Which communication style did Gabe use to reset the interaction?
3. What is the likely outcome?

The Pearsons continue to favor a partnership with Gabe and Dr. O'Brien. This time, Gabe meets the Pearsons where they are by using a partner communication style. As a result, Gabe fully elicits the Pearsons' concerns and relays them to Dr. O'Brien, who provides a clear diagnosis, educates the Pearsons, and involves them in shared decision-making. The Pearsons appear more satisfied with the visit.

Adapt Communication Styles to the Team

Communication Styles

Expert

Expert practice leaders tend to move forward with their agenda, assume their colleagues' values are the same as theirs, prioritize practice productivity, and set goals for the veterinary team. The expert communication style is prevalent among veterinary practice leaders who demonstrate a more coercive style, leading the practice team with their initiatives. Without an opportunity for the team to voice their opinion, colleagues may feel undervalued, disempowered, not invested, and unmotivated. As a result, they may not speak up with creative ideas or alternative viewpoints.

Partner

Partner practice leaders value collaboration, invite the contributions of others, strive for buy-in, and foster a healthy workplace culture. A partner capitalizes on the collective wisdom of their team to problem-solve and brainstorm alternative solutions. Partners embrace, recognize, and value their colleagues' expertise, such as their specialized technical and professional skills, accumulated knowledge and experiences, day to day practice successes and challenges, and individual ideas, beliefs, and values. By using the team's wealth of knowledge, more creative and diverse solutions come to fruition.

As with clients, when colleague communication styles are aligned, more positive outcomes prevail. When styles are discordant, desired outcomes are not achieved, impacting the practice, veterinary team, clients, patients, and ourselves. Engage individual team members and coordinate the team by assessing and matching communication styles (Sidebar 2.5).

Sidebar 2.5   Improved Team Outcomes of Aligning Communication Styles

Empower individual engagement
Foster team engagement
Promote team coordination
Encourage team buy-in
Increase accuracy
Enhance efficiency
Enrich self-fulfillment
Cultivate job satisfaction
Achieve staff retention

Be Flexible

In team interactions, communication styles are highly dynamic. Like client interactions, we need to pull off being a "relationship ninja," adapting to what the situation requires of us. Returning to Figure 2.1 urgency also drives the use of communication styles in colleague-to-colleague interactions. Assume the expert role when an employee's or patient's safety is at risk, to guide them out of danger. Once out of harm's way, partner with the colleague in a meeting to discuss changes to protocols to prevent future occurrences.

Another example is engaging with a highly emotional – angry, frustrated, anxious – colleague. Initially, in an expert role, we might invite them to sit in our office, take a walk, or reflect overnight. Once settled, we switch to partnering to elicit the colleague's perspective and invite them to share the story underlying the strong emotions to form a collaborative plan for moving forward successfully.

Commonly Asked Questions Related to Team Communication Styles

How Can I Be a Practice Leader and a Partner at the Same Time? They Seem Antagonistic to Each Other

Some veterinary leaders view partnership-building as wishy-washy or lacking clear, strong leadership. It is difficult to relinquish control and let colleagues take the reins and run with their ideas. Practice leaders may feel left out, anxious, fearful, or helpless.

In collaborative relationships, leaders maintain their role as practice owner, manager, veterinarian, lead technician, or client service supervisor. In striving for cooperation, the practice leader engages colleagues in a dialogue in which both parties bring their expertise to the discussion. The partner-facilitator elicits and respects their colleagues' input; invites them to share their perspectives, knowledge and skillsets, and relevant background information; and, finally, offers their own concerns, thoughts, and viewpoints. The result is a meeting of experts, capitalizing on the strengths of everyone, and openness to see other's perspective or change our ideas.

As previously acknowledged in this chapter, although the partner style takes more time up front, the rewards are substantial and long-lasting. Over time, the efficiency of the group's decision-making process improves; our colleagues benefit from their voices being heard, and because all parties are investing in the plan moving forward, the practice enjoys strong staff retention. It is a win-win in the end: good for the individuals and good for the team.

How Do I Find Time to Achieve Buy-In with the Team?

How do we find the time? We make it a priority and consider it an investment for short-term and long-term rewards. Achieving buy-in requires eliciting the full agenda early on to gather expectations. Take time to explore where colleagues are coming from, and value their thoughts and feelings, knowledge levels, backgrounds, and skillsets. Understanding our colleagues' concerns, priorities, and perspectives enables us to often tailor the conversation to incorporate their needs; this accelerates the decision-making process and promotes buy-in.

In addition, assess each colleague's communication style, depth and breadth of knowledge, and information preferences to formulate a targeted message. Knowing how to do this eliminates those seemingly endless meetings in which too much time is spent presenting information that everyone already knows, discussing options no one wants, or clarifying and untangling all kinds of preventable miscommunications. Investing time in our colleagues early on prevents wasting time later.

Team Scenario

Set the Scene: Marta, the client service supervisor, who prefers brainstorming, is meeting with Theresa, the authoritative, no-nonsense practice owner, to discuss concerns about client and patient congestion at the front desk.

> **THERESA:**   *Hi, Marta. What do you want to talk about?*
>
> **MARTA:**   *Thanks for meeting with me today. I'd like to work together to come up with solutions for the congestion at the front desk, which seems to be getting worse and worse.*
>
> **THERESA:**   *Well, the only solution I see is hiring another client service coordinator, and I can tell you right now that we can't afford it.*
>
> **MARTA:**   *Yes. Listen, we've got long wait times for clients, and callers are put on hold for five minutes or longer. Yesterday, while their caregivers were waiting to check out, two dogs got into a fight, and a woman with a stressed cat got flustered, canceled her appointment, and walked out. This is impacting our whole practice.*
>
> **THERESA:**   *Given our budget, we're just going to have to make do with the current team. You are the client service supervisor, and I hope you and your team come up with a solution. Go to it!*
>
> **MARTA:**   *I will. Thanks for making the time!*

Before reading on, reflect on the following three questions:

1. Which communication style is Marta favoring?
2. Which communication style is Theresa using?
3. What is the likely outcome?

Recovery Team Scenario

Set the Scene: In the previous scenario, Marta attempted to use the partner style to gain Theresa's attention, with little result. Theresa, as an expert, was down-to-business and looking for answers. Because of the misalignment, Theresa became frustrated and abruptly called the meeting to an end, and Marta conceded and departed the meeting without solutions.

A week passed since Marta and Theresa last spoke about the congestion problem at the front desk. This time, Theresa, the practice owner, asks to sit down with Marta, the client service supervisor, to revisit her concerns.

> **THERESA:** *Thank you for meeting with me last week, Marta. I apologize. I was super-stressed and didn't hear you out as you deserved. Also, I got complaints from more clients this week. I had no idea the congestion problem had gotten so bad! So, if you are willing, I'd like to revisit our conversation.*
>
> **MARTA:** *Thank you, Theresa. I appreciate that. I'd like to work with you to come up with potential approaches and solutions.*
>
> **THERESA:** *Me too. What do you think is the source of the problem?*
>
> **MARTA:** *It seems like the front-desk congestion may be symptomatic of our growing caseload.*
>
> **THERESA:** *Sounds like our caseload is exceeding our staffing. What are your thoughts on how we can address the issue?*
>
> **MARTA:** *I'd like to discuss the challenges with my team and come up with some options for your consideration.*
>
> **THERESA:** *That's reasonable. I know that hiring another client service coordinator will come up, and I am not sure that fits within our budget. Could you work with them to identify other solutions as well?*
>
> **MARTA:** *Sure. We will likely need to take a two-pronged approach: one that addresses client frustrations and the other that prevents staff stress.*
>
> **THERESA:** *How about we start with outlining solutions to our clients' current frustrations, and then we can look at how each solution may impact the client service team before making a final decision?*
>
> **MARTA:** *That sounds like a reasonable place to start.*

Before reading on, again, reflect on the following three questions:

1. Which communication style is Marta favoring?
2. Which communication style did Theresa use to reset the interaction?
3. What is the likely outcome?

Marta continues to pursue the conversation favoring a partner style. Theresa requests a follow-up meeting, apologizes, and elicits Marta's agenda, concerns, and ideas transitioning to a partner style to reset the interaction. By aligning styles, they work collaboratively to move forward in solving the client congestion problem, increasing the likelihood of finding a solution the entire team will invest in.

Put the Communication Styles into Practice

For the following exercises, refer to Figure 2.1, which depicts the four communication styles (expert-in-charge to facilitator) applicable for interacting with clients and colleagues. As a review, experts take the lead, drive their agenda, and shot-put information, leaving little room for the contributions of others. Partners strive for collaboration and reciprocity and Frisbee information back and forth to elicit perspectives, contributions, and feedback from others.

Do-It-Yourself Exercises

Exercise 2.1   Skill Spot – Communication Styles

For each of the following client and colleague statements, indicate whether it represents the expert or partner communication style.

1. *We will work together to develop the best plan for you and Titus.*

2. *Marta, I think you should hire another client service coordinator.*

3. *I'd like to examine Titus's eye, do a tear test, and check for a scratch on the outside of his eye.*

4. *Marta, let's gather the team to see what ideas they bring to address these challenges.*

Exercise 2.2   Self-Reflect – Client Communication Styles

Depending on your practice role, reflect on your client interactions. The first step is to understand your natural communication style. The next is to assess the style favored by the client you are working with and then adapt your style to theirs in the moment. This may require expanding your repertoire and developing an approach that is in direct contrast to the one that feels most natural to you.

1. Put a star on the Communication Styles graph in Figure 2.1 to indicate your natural habitat. What is the style you use most commonly?

2. Put an asterisk on the graph to mark the style you use when stressed or under pressure.

3. Reflect on a recent client challenge. What was your client's communication style?

4. What verbal and nonverbal cues did you pick up on from yourself or your client to determine whether your style was aligned with that of your client? Generate a list of one or two nonverbal cues and one or two verbal cues you observed.

5. How can you adapt your communication style when your client favors a style that is not natural to you? What can you do or say in the moment to get in alignment? Write down three ideas.

Exercise 2.3   Self-Reflect – Colleague Communication Styles

Now, take what you learned about your communication style with clients and apply it to your direct team.

1. Reflect on individuals on your immediate team or in the practice, and consider the preferred communication styles of three to five colleagues you regularly interact with. Plot their names and styles on Figure 2.1.

2. Consider recent interactions with these colleagues, and choose one interaction to explore in more depth.

3. For the interaction you identified, follow these steps:

   a. What was your communication style?

   b. What communication style did your colleague favor?

   c. What word would you use to characterize the interaction for yourself and for your colleague (e.g. awkward, tense, relaxed, satisfying, or mutual)?

   d. What verbal and nonverbal cues did you pick up from yourself or your colleague that indicated the interaction was aligned?

   e. What enabled you to meet and align with your colleague's communication style? Or how might you do so in the future?

   f. When **not** aligned with your colleague's communication style, how might you adjust your approach to meet that of your colleague? Create one or two concrete verbal phrases or nonverbal behaviors that would align your approach with your colleague's communication style.

Engage-the-Entire-Team Exercises

Exercise 2.4   Learn Your Team's Communication Styles

Bring your team together to teach lessons from this chapter, explore their communication style preferences, and create greater awareness of communication styles among colleagues. If conducting the exercise with your entire practice team, you might break into groups of four or five individuals who work closely together.

1. To get everyone on the same page, introduce the group to descriptions of the expert (i.e. shot-put) and partner (i.e. Frisbee) communication styles:

   a. On a whiteboard or flipchart, as a group, brainstorm advantages and disadvantages of the expert and partner communication styles.

   b. Present Figure 2.1, and locate the expert and partner communication styles on the graph.

2. Ask everyone to reflect and identify their "natural habitat" or preferred communication style on the graph using the following questions:

   a. *What is your go-to communication style?*

   b. *How does that communication style work for you (i.e. strengths)?*

   c. *What can be challenging about that communication style for you (i.e. struggles)?*

3. In small groups who work together closely, take turns inviting each team member to share their identified communication style, along with the strengths and challenges identified:

   a. Review the composition of communication styles within the group.

b. Discuss examples of when the working group's communication styles work well together.

c. Provide examples of when the working group's communication styles present challenges.

d. Moving forward, identify how each individual's approach might differ depending on the communication style of the other person by posing these questions:

    i. *What might you do less of?*

    ii. *What might you do more of?*

Exercise 2.5   Debrief Team Scenarios

As a follow-up to the previous exercise, bring your team together to debrief various team decision-making scenarios that were challenging and determine what communication style(s) were used and the resulting outcome. If conducting the exercise with your entire practice team, you might break into groups of four or five individuals.

1. Create a list of recent challenging team-based decision-making scenarios, and assign one to each small group.

2. Ask the small groups to reflect on the decision-making process: led by an expert or a partner? What were the resulting outcomes?

3. Work through the following questions to guide the small-group discussions:

    a. *Thinking back on that situation, how was the decision made (i.e. "told" or "worked together")?*

    b. *What role did you play? What role would you have liked to play?*

    c. *What were the positive and challenging outcomes of the decision?*

    d. *If you had to do it all over again, what would you do or want done differently?*

4. Take the lessons learned, and project forward to anticipated decisions that lie ahead for the team.

5. Choose two upcoming projects, and assign them to the small groups.

6. Work through the following set of questions to guide the small-group discussions:

    a. *What are the importance, objectives, and intended impact of the project?*

    b. *Who should be involved in the decision-making?*

    c. *What is the urgency of the decision?*

    d. *What is the appropriate communication style to get there?*

    e. *What can be applied from past lessons to this project?*

    f. *What are the desired outcomes for each individual involved?*

    g. *What might be the required trade offs in desired outcomes?*

    h. *How will the group or team move forward with the project?*

7. Close this exercise by first allowing time for personal reflection on the following question and then inviting each team member to share their commitments out loud:

    a. *When communication styles are **not** in alignment, how, in the moment, will you respectfully ask for what you need? What would that sound like?*

Take It Away

1. Effective communication starts with knowing and identifying **your personal communication style** during routine and stressful interactions with clients or colleagues.

    a. With the **expert communication style**, you take the lead, and your client or colleague plays a more passive role.

    b. With the **partner communication style**, you invite clients' or colleagues' perspectives and contributions and take them into account during agenda-setting, decision-making, and problem-solving.

2. Next, develop an awareness of and appreciation for the **communication style of others.**

3. Finally, be completely present in the conversation to assess whether **communication styles are aligned**. If not, reset the interaction by apologizing, requesting to start over, and making adjustments to meet clients or colleagues where they are.

Answer Key

Exercise 2.1   Skill-Spot – Communication Styles

1. *We will work together to develop the best plan for you and Titus.* [partner]

2. *Marta, I think you should hire another client service coordinator.* [expert]

3. *I'd like to examine Titus's eye, do a tear test, and check for a scratch on the outside of his eye.* [expert]

4. *Marta, let's gather the team to see what ideas they bring to address these challenges.* [partner]

References

Barbour, A. (2000). *Making Contact or Making Sense: Functional and Dysfunctional Ways of Relating,* Humanities Institute Lecture 1999–2000 Series. Colorado: University of Denver.

Coe, J.B., Adams, C.L., and Bonnett, B.N. (2008). A focus group study of veterinarians' and pet owners' perceptions of veterinarian–client communication in companion animal practice. *J. Am. Vet. Med. Assoc.* 233 (7): 1072–1080. https://doi.org/10.2460/javma.233.7.1072.

Janke, N., Coe, J.B., Bernardo, T.M. et al. (2021). Pet owners' and veterinarians' perceptions of information exchange and clinical decision-making in companion animal practice. *PLoS ONE* 16 (2): e0245632. https://doi.org/10.1371/journal.pone.0245632.

Kurtz, S., Silverman, J., and Draper, J. (2005). *Teaching and Learning Communication Skills in Medicine.* London, England: CRC Press.

Lussier, M.T. and Richard, C. (2008). Because one shoe doesn't fit all: a repertoire of doctor–patient relationships. *Can. Fam. Physic.* 54 (8): 1089–1092.

Moore, I.C., Coe, J.B., Adams, C.L. et al. (2014). The role of veterinary team effectiveness in job satisfaction and burnout in companion animal veterinary clinics. *J. Am. Vet. Med. Assoc.* 245 (5): 513–524. https://doi.org/10.2460/javma.245.5.513.

Moore, I.C., Coe, J.B., Adams, C.L. et al. (2015). Exploring the impact of toxic attitudes and a toxic environment on the veterinary healthcare team. *Front. Vet. Sci.* 2: 78. https://doi.org/10.3389/fvets.2015.00078.

Nogueira Borden, L.J., Adams, C.L., Bonnett, B.N. et al. (2010). Use of the measure of patient-centered communication to analyze euthanasia discussions in companion animal practice. *J. Am. Vet. Med. Assoc.* 237 (11): 1275–1286. https://doi.org/10.2460/javma.237.11.1275.

Pizzolon, C., Coe, J.B., and Shaw, J.R. (2019). Evaluation of team effectiveness and personal empathy for associations with professional quality of life and job satisfaction in companion animal practice personnel. *J. Am. Vet. Med. Assoc.* 245 (10): 513–524. https://doi.org/10.2460/javma.254.10.1204.

Roter, D.L. (2000). The enduring and evolving nature of the patient–physician relationship. *Patient Educ. Couns.* 39 (1): 5–15. https://doi: 10.1016/s0738-3991(99)00086-5.

Shaw, J.R., Bonnett, B.N., Adams, C.L., and Roter, D.L. (2006). Veterinarian–client–patient communication patterns used during clinical appointments in companion animal practice. *J. Am. Vet. Med. Assoc.* 228 (5): 714–721. https://doi.org/10.2460/javma.228.5.714.

Shaw, J.R., Bonnett, B.N., Adams, C.L. et al. (2008). Veterinarian–client–patient communication during wellness appointments versus appointments related to a health problem in companion animal practice. *J. Am. Vet. Med. Assoc.* 233 (10): 1576–1586. https://doi.org/10.2460/javma.233.10.1576.

Shaw, J.R., Bonnett, B.N., Roter, D.L. et al. (2012). Gender differences in veterinarian–client–patient communication in companion animal practice. *J. Am. Vet. Med. Assoc.* 241 (1): 81–88. https://doi.org/10.2460/javma.241.1.81.

3

Opening-the-Interaction

Abstract

We do not get a second chance to make a first impression with a client or a colleague. There are multiple opportunities to impact client experiences every day. From the initial phone call, to walking into the clinic, to meeting and interacting with the veterinary team, to concluding the visit, every exchange contributes to the client's satisfaction with and confidence and trust in the veterinary practice. In this chapter, we introduce three communication skills – preparation, introduction, and agenda-setting – to get the visit with a client or meeting with a colleague off to the right start. Agenda-setting is an instrumental communication skill at the beginning of every appointment or meeting. The client's or colleague's agenda is revealed through question-asking up front to fully elicit the reasons for the interaction, including concerns, goals, expectations, and priorities. Establishing the agenda at the start of the visit or meeting paves the way for collaborative planning throughout the rest of the interaction. With the client's or colleague's agenda in mind, we create a tailored plan.

SELF-ASSESSMENT QUESTIONS

1. What kind of first impression do I make at the beginning of an interaction?
2. How do I elicit my client's or colleague's agenda up front, including their reasons for the visit or meeting, concerns, goals, expectations, and priorities?
3. How do I meld my client's or colleague's priorities with mine to establish a mutually agreed-on agenda?

Introduction

We do not get a second chance to make a first impression with a client or a colleague. In a veterinary practice, there are multiple opportunities to impact client experiences every day. From their initial phone call, to walking into the clinic, to meeting and interacting with the veterinary team, to concluding the visit; every exchange contributes to the client's satisfaction with and trust and confidence in the veterinary practice team (Sidebar 3.1).

Sidebar 3.1   Clinical Outcomes of an Effective Opening

Build relationship
Foster satisfaction
Enhance efficiency
Provide structure
Nurture confidence

The client's first impression of the veterinary practice often starts online while viewing the website, looking at reviews, or scheduling an appointment. The client's assessment continues with the initial telephone conversation and in-person interaction with the client service representative or coordinator at the reception desk, followed by the veterinary technician's welcome, and finally the veterinarian's greeting on entering the examination room. These touchpoints set the stage for all that follows.

The opening is a critical time to make a positive impression, put an anxious client or fearful patient at ease, diffuse frustrations, reassure a panicked client in an emergency, or comfort a tearful client. These deceptively simple exchanges set up the conversation for success – and likewise for failure. So, ensure that the entire team, especially at the reception desk, is well-staffed and trained to make warm connections with clients.

Friendly openings are just as important for engaging with colleagues as they are for clients. Use common salutations to welcome job interviewees, greet colleagues as they arrive to work, and acknowledge attendees at the start of a meeting. Doing so sets a supportive tone for subsequent conversations and nurtures successful professional relationships.

In this chapter, we explore three key communication skills to begin an interaction with a client or colleague: preparation, introduction, and agenda-setting (Sidebar 3.2). We provide examples in two locations: the examination room, working with Mr. Dolohov and his rabbit, Francis; and the treatment room (Hunter and Shaw 2011), welcoming Jill Fritz, a prospective new employee visiting the practice for a day-long working interview.

Sidebar 3.2   Three Communication Skills for Opening-the-Interaction

Preparation
Introduction
Agenda-setting

Set the Scene

Client Scenario: Mr. Dolohov presents on time for his appointment with Francis, a two-year-old, male-castrated, lop-eared rabbit that is losing weight. Unfortunately, the schedule is running 20 minutes behind. On top of that, Francis was originally scheduled with Dr. Morrison, his regular veterinarian; but Dr. Morrison was called into an emergency, so Francis will be seen by Dr. Hernandez. The appointment is clearly not getting off to a good start.

Team Scenario: Meanwhile, Jill Fritz, a registered veterinary technician, arrived for her day-long onsite job interview with team members Mario, Sharma, and Andrea.

Stepping into Dr. Hernandez's and Mario's, Sharma's, and Andrea's shoes, self-reflect on:

1. How would I open the appointment with Mr. Dolohov to make amends and put him at ease?
2. How would I put my best foot forward in welcoming Jill?

Opening Client Interactions

Key Communication Skills for Opening-the-Interaction

Preparation

Definition
Taking time to mentally prepare for the interaction.

Technique
Preparation may be as short as taking a breath between appointments or consciously stepping aside to clear our mind of our to-do list and shifting our focus to the task or client at hand. There may not be enough time to fully prepare, and even a short break sets us straight. Take time to review the patient's medical record and previous medical history to enhance continuity of care and communication. If time runs out, be transparent and ask the client to fill in the blanks: for example, *Unfortunately, I didn't have an opportunity to review Francis's record. Can you share what's been going on?*

Introduction

Definition
An act of respect and etiquette where we formally present ourselves to others, including exchanging names and niceties, and clarifying roles.

Technique
The introduction is composed of **five steps** (Sidebar 3.3).

Sidebar 3.3   Five Steps of the Introduction

1. Make an introduction to the client(s), and clarify your role.
2. Make an introduction to the pet(s).
3. Invite the client(s) to introduce themselves and their pet(s).
4. Demonstrate interest in the client(s) and their pet(s).
5. Address any immediate concern(s) right away.

Step 1: Make an introduction to the client(s), and clarify your role.
Enter the examination room with a warm greeting, a welcoming gesture if appropriate, solid eye contact, and clearly state your name and your pronouns. Inform the client of your role in their pet's care or role within the veterinary clinic. Make introductions with every individual in the examination room.

Step 2: Make an introduction to the pet(s).
Allow the pet(s) to present, or locate the pet(s) in the room and address them. The order of introductions may vary based on whether the client or pet approaches first in the examination room. The pet may come up and initiate a greeting before you engage with the client.

Step 3: Invite the client(s) to introduce themselves and their pet(s).
Ask the client to share how they would like to be addressed, which invites the correct pronunciation of client and pet name(s) and an opportunity to identify accurate pronouns.

Step 4: Demonstrate interest in the client(s) and their pet(s).
Depending on the context, explore the trip to the clinic or make social chitchat to establish initial rapport. Good conversation starters include a personal connection, current events, weather, sports, or the personality, name, breed, or composition of the pet.

Step 5: Address any immediate concern(s) right away.
These may include presenting emotions, such as sadness, anxiety, frustration, or anger; the doctor running late; or a change in the expected doctor.

Examples
Veterinary technician: *Hello, Mr. Dolohov. I'm Lindsey,* [make introduction to the client] *the veterinary technician working with Dr. Hernandez and I use she/her pronouns.* [clarify your role] *This must be Francis.* [make introduction to pet] *He's so cute!* [demonstrate interest in client and pet] *You were expecting to see Dr. Morrison today. Unfortunately, he's tied up in an emergency.* [address immediate concern(s)] *Would it be all right if Dr. Hernandez sees Francis today?*

Veterinarian: *Hello, Mr. Dolohov. I'm Dr. Hernandez.* [clarify your role] *You can call me Vanessa and I use she/her pronouns.* [make introduction to the client] *It's nice to meet you! I joined the practice last year, and I've heard great things about you and Francis from Dr. Morrison.* [demonstrate interest in client and pet] *I'm sorry I kept you waiting.* [address immediate concern(s)]

Agenda-Setting

Definition
A series of steps leading to a mutually agreed-on task list for the appointment. The agenda is revealed through a question-asking process at the beginning of the appointment to fully elicit the client's reason(s) for the visit, concerns for their pet, and goals, expectations, and priorities. This complete laundry list of issues, procedures, and topics ordered by priority formulates the topics to explore in the history and creates a structured plan for the appointment. Agenda-setting incorporates both the client's and veterinary team's agendas and creates a roadmap for the visit, so it is crucial to take time up front for this process.

Technique
Agenda-setting is composed of **six steps** (Sidebar 3.4).

Sidebar 3.4 Six Steps to Agenda-Setting

1. Elicit your client's agenda:
   a. Reason(s) for the visit
   b. Client concerns for the pet
   c. Goals, expectations, and priorities.
2. Summarize the client's agenda.
3. Check for remaining items.
4. Offer your (i.e., the veterinary professional's) agenda items.
5. Negotiate a mutual agenda.
6. Summarize the mutually agreed-on agenda.

Step 1: Elicit your client's agenda.

a. Reason(s) for the visit: Why the individual requested the appointment, which often constitutes the presenting complaint(s).

> ***What*** *brings you and Francis in today?* [reasons]

b. Client concerns for the pet: Worries, anxieties, or trepidations regarding the pet.

> ***What*** *other concerns do you have?* [concerns]

c. Goals, expectations, and priorities: What they would like to achieve or accomplish during the interaction, and what is most urgent or important to them.

> ***What*** *are your goals for today's visit?* [goals]
> ***What*** *are you hoping we can do for you and Francis today?* [expectations]
> ***How*** *would you like to prioritize our time together?* [priorities]

To elicit the client's agenda, use open-ended inquiry (e.g. questions that start with *Tell me, Explain, Describe, Share, What, or How*) to explore the breadth of topics. Open-ended inquiry invites clients to share all their concerns. So as not to sound redundant, we build a set of open-ended agenda-setting questions to elicit our client's full agenda (Box 3.1). No matter what is written in the appointment book, take time to understand the client's full agenda, since priorities may change since they scheduled their appointment. Gather the reason(s) for the visit, explore the client's concerns for their pet, and obtain their goals, expectations, and priorities.

Box 3.1   Build a Repertoire of Agenda-Setting Inquiries

What else would you like to discuss with Dr. Hernandez? [reasons]
What else would you like to focus on during our conversation? [reasons]

Share with me what worries you about Francis. [concerns]
What is going on with Francis that concerns you? [concerns]

How can we address your objectives? [goals]
Describe what you would like to accomplish today. [goals]

Tell me what you expect from us today. [expectations]
How can we best help you and Francis? [expectations]

Elaborate on what is most important to you. [priorities]
What is your number-one priority for today's visit? [priorities]

Clients often express more than one concern to discuss with their veterinary professional or veterinarian (Dysart et al. 2011) (Research Spotlight 3.1). Use these findings as a litmus test and motivation to continue to check for any remaining agenda items and try to obtain at least three or four items for discussion (Beckman and Frankel 1984). While it may seem formulaic to elicit a client's agenda by asking numerous questions in a row, the client may come up with yet another item for discussion. Each question type takes a different angle and obtains a discrete response. Agenda-setting protects against making assumptions about why the client set the appointment or what they would like to achieve.

Research Spotlight 3.1

Closed vs. Open-Ended Solicitation of Client Concerns

In a study of veterinarians' solicitation of client concerns at the beginning of the visit, veterinarians actively solicited clients' concerns in only 37% of the appointments studied (Dysart et al. 2011). Using an open-ended approach to eliciting client concerns at the beginning of the visit revealed a significantly greater number of client concerns than using a closed-ended approach. These findings emphasize the importance of using open-ended inquiry at the beginning of the visit to elicit a client's agenda.

Open-ended solicitation	Closed-ended solicitation
No concern – 24% (22/93)	No concern – 60% (18/30)
1 concern – 65% (60/93)	1 concern – 27% (8/30)
≥2 concerns – 11% (10/93)	2 concerns – 13% (4/30)

Step 2: Summarize the client's agenda.
After eliciting the client's agenda, review or list the agenda items (i.e., reason(s) for the visit, client's concerns for their pet, and their goals, expectations, and priorities) to ensure that they are accurate and inclusive.

> *You're concerned that Francis continues to **lose weight** and he's **not responding** to the treatment. So, you're interested in taking a **different tack** because you're worried that he does not have much body reserves left.* [summarize client's agenda]

Step 3: Check for remaining items by continuing to use open-ended inquiry, being exhaustive to discover all the client's concerns, goals, expectations, and priorities.

> ***What** else would you like to discuss today?* [check]
> ***What** would you like to add?* [check]

It is challenging to stick only to agenda-setting until complete. Be mindful of being lured and delving deeper into problems as they are revealed. Going down the information-gathering rabbit hole too early is precarious, as it prevents discovering all the client's agenda items. This puts the appointment at risk for an "oh, by the way" moment at the end of the interview (Research Spotlight 3.2). If the client leads by providing history, redirect: *I would like to hear more about that. Before doing so, I want to make sure I've heard all of your concerns.*

Research Spotlight 3.2

"Oh, By the Way"

When veterinarians did not actively solicit client concerns at the beginning of an appointment, the client was four times more likely to raise an issue at the end of the visit (Dysart et al. 2011). Late-arising concerns at the end of the visit – also known as "doorknob issues" – reduce appointment efficiency, compromise client satisfaction, and increase stress on the veterinary team. These results highlight that it pays to take time up front to fully elicit the client's agenda, to prevent "oh, by the way" moments arising at the end of the appointment.

Step 4: Offer your (i.e., the veterinary professional's) agenda items to discuss alongside those of the client.

> *I'm concerned that Francis's teeth may be the culprit, so I'd like to get a better **look in his mouth** today. Also, I'd like to explore Francis's **diet** in greater detail.* [offer veterinary professional's agenda]

Step 5: Negotiate a mutual agenda.
The veterinary professional may view the importance or prioritization of the agenda items differently from the client, or there may not be enough time to address all the agenda items.

> *Let's start with exploring Francis' **weight loss**, what you've tried, and how he's responded.* [client's agenda] *Then, I am going to suggest we sedate Francis to take a **good look in his mouth**.* [veterinary professional's agenda] *Would you be willing to leave him with us for the afternoon, so I have time to do so? After I have had a good look in his mouth, I will give you a call, and we can discuss **alternative treatments**.* [client's agenda] *What are your thoughts about this plan for moving forward?*

Step 6: Summarize the mutually agreed-on agenda.
Meld your agenda with that of the client, and summarize the shared approach for how to move forward and structure the appointment.

> *So, we agreed to start by digging deeper to determine why Francis continues to **lose weight despite treatment**.* [client's agenda] *We'll investigate his **diet**, and you will leave him with us this afternoon so I can thoroughly **examine Francis's mouth**.* [veterinary professional's agenda] *Then I will call you, and we can discuss options for a **different approach**.* [client's agenda] *What have I missed?* [check]

Outcomes of Agenda-Setting

With a mutually agreed-on map in hand, we are well-positioned to meet or exceed our client's expectations, engendering confidence and client satisfaction. Establishing the agenda at the beginning of the visit also paves the way for collaborative planning in the second half of the appointment. Knowing the client's agenda, we create a tailored plan that tightly aligns with the client's goals, expectations, and priorities. When the diagnostic or treatment plan is a good fit for the client and patient, the client is more likely to adhere to and invest in it.

If it is not possible to meet the client's agenda fully or in part, we negotiate an alternate route early on to enhance appointment efficiency: delegate tasks, request a drop-off, or schedule a follow-up visit. Essentially, the agenda keeps the veterinary team and client on the same path; without it, it is easy to get lost.

Agenda-Setting Is a Veterinary Team Sport

Agenda-setting starts with the client service coordinator or representative identifying the initial agenda during appointment scheduling. This evolves when the veterinary technician elicits additional items, and it is confirmed by the veterinarian, who summarizes the final agenda with the client. Everyone plays an integral role in inviting more concerns and ensuring that the agenda is complete, thorough, and accurate (Box 3.2).

Box 3.2   Agenda-Setting Is a Veterinary Team Sport

1. **Client service coordinator or representative**

   a. Gathers the initial agenda (i.e. reason(s), concerns, goals, priorities, and expectations) during appointment scheduling.

   b. Notes the agenda items in the medical record.

2. **Veterinary technician**

   a. Summarizes to the client the agenda captured in the medical record by the client service coordinator or representative and checks for new arising items.

   *I see in my notes that Francis is here for continued **weight loss**. You're concerned that the **treatments aren't working** and are hoping for **another solution**. [summarize client's agenda] What else would you like to cover today? [check]*

   b. If the agenda is missing from the record, gather the initial agenda directly (i.e. reason(s), concerns, goals, priorities, and expectations).

   c. Summarizes the agenda when presenting the case to the veterinarian.

   *Dr. Hernandez, the reason for Francis's visit is **weight loss**. Mr. Dolohov is concerned that Francis is **continuing to lose weight despite treatment**, and his goal is to find out what's going on and try a **new approach** to the problem. [summarize client's agenda]*

3. **Veterinarian**

   a. Clarifies and confirms the client's agenda with the veterinary technician before entering the exam room.

   *Thanks for filling me in, Lindsey <veterinary technician>. So, Mr. Dolohov and Francis are here for **continued weight loss** with **no response to previous treatments**, and he wants a **different approach**. [summarize client's agenda] What am I missing? [check]*

   b. In the exam room, reflects the agenda back to the client and checks for any additional agenda items.

   *Lindsey shared with me that Francis is here for **continued weight loss**. You're concerned that he's **not responding to treatment** so far, and your goals for today are to **identify other ways** for Francis to gain weight. [summarize client's agenda] How else can I help you and Francis today? [check]*

Commonly Asked Questions Related to Opening-the-Interaction

How Can I Request a Second Chance at the Opening?

At times, the opening of the appointment is rushed and full of distractions, which results in missing the chance to build rapport or identify a client's red flags. Getting it right entails taking a breath, slowing down, and being fully present to accurately read the situation. We will not always get it right and cannot expect perfection from ourselves or others. So, when the opening gets botched, apologize to the client, express a desire to make it right, and request a reset.

I'm sorry. I didn't get the opportunity to greet you and Francis as I'd like. I'm Sherry, [make introduction to the client] one of the client service coordinators and I use she/her pronouns. [clarify your role] I apologize for the wait and that we did not let you know ahead of time that we are running behind. [address immediate concern(s)] Can I get you a coffee?

How Do I Address Clients Who Are on Their Cell Phones?

In today's world of expanding technologies and widespread internet access, this will happen. The first step is to take a deep breath and leave assumptions at the door. It is easy to become frustrated and feel that clients are wasting our time. For the client, this may be an important call: possibly a family emergency, a sick child who needs to be picked up at school, or an attempt to keep a partner who could not attend the veterinary visit well-informed.

Take a minute to check in with clients on their cell phones during appointments. Give them the benefit of the doubt that their intention was not to be disrespectful. Invite them to share what might be going on, determine whether to redirect their attention, or inquire further about how to be of assistance. Preempt this socially awkward situation with a poster in the reception area that reminds clients to silence their cell phones. Even so, a client may take a call.

> *I see you are on the phone. Would you like to take a minute before we start?*
>
> *I see you need to take a call. Would you like to reschedule our appointment?*
>
> *That seems important, so I'll give you some privacy and return in 5 or 10 minutes.*

If the phone call is not critical or urgent, and the client persists, gently break in to request the client's attention, offer to attend to their needs, and request to get started.

> *Sorry to interrupt. I want to make sure we have enough time together. Could you take that call later, so we can start our appointment?*
>
> *Excuse me. With a full appointment schedule this afternoon, I want to be sure to give you and Francis the time you deserve. May we begin?*
>
> *I'm sorry – we're almost finished. Would you mind taking that call later?*

Routine Client Scenario

Set the Scene: Lindsey, the veterinary technician, gathers Mr. Dolohov's agenda and relays to Dr. Hernandez that his primary concern is Francis's weight.

Preparation: In the hallway, Dr. Hernandez and Lindsey review the case together and discuss offering Mr. Dolohov the option of dropping off Francis for the afternoon to allow adequate time for an oral examination under sedation. Then Dr. Hernandez enters the examination room.

Introduction:

> *Thank you for your patience; I'm sorry that we've kept you waiting.* [address immediate concern(s)] *I'm Dr. Hernandez and I use she/her pronouns.* [make introduction to the client] *Dr. Morrison asked me to step in to take care of you and Francis today* [clarify your role]. *It's a pleasure to meet you both.* [demonstrate interest in client and pet]

Agenda-setting:

> *Lindsey shared that you're worried about Francis's **weight loss and lack of response to treatment** and are hoping for a **different plan**.* [summarize client's agenda] *What else would you like to cover?* [check]
>
> *I'd also like to get a full history of what's been going on with Francis.* [veterinary professional's agenda]

> *I'm going to need more time to take a good look in Francis's mouth. Would you be willing to leave Francis with us for the afternoon?* [veterinary professional's agenda]
>
> *After I examine Francis's mouth, I'll schedule a time for us to talk later this afternoon about a plan for moving forward* [summarize the mutually agreed-on agenda].

Challenging Client Scenario

Set the Scene: Dr. Hernandez enters the examination room, and Mr. Dolohov is on his cell phone and continues to talk despite her presence. With appointments piling up due to the walk-in emergency, Dr. Hernandez's stress level is mounting.

Preparation: Dr. Hernandez listens patiently for a moment, takes a deep breath and then respectfully interjects and introduces herself.

Introduction:

> *Excuse me for interrupting. I'm Dr. Hernandez,* [make introduction to the client], *and I use she/her pronouns. I will be caring for Francis today.* [clarify your role] *It sounds like the person on the other end of the phone is worried about Francis.* [address immediate concern(s)]
>
> *I'm wondering if they might like to join our appointment. We can put them on speakerphone. That way, we can get started, they'll have an opportunity to be involved, and I can hear their thoughts about Francis as well.*
>
> *If they do not have time, would it be all right if you called them back later when we know more?*

Talk through Technology – Telephone Communication

This book focuses predominantly on verbal face-to-face communication with our clients and colleagues. However, equally important are verbal communication at a distance and written communication. Consider the ways we converse with clients outside the examination room: on the telephone or video call; discharge statements, client handouts, or client forms; text, email, and social media messages; and online reviews and responses. In the Talk through Technology sections of the chapters that follow, we dig deeper into each form of communication and offer tips for successful communication. The good news is that the same communication principles and skills apply.

How we manage these interactions builds or breaks down relationships and reputations. The first personal introduction to the veterinary practice is often over the telephone, so it is critical to consider what messages are sent during this initial contact. First impressions are lasting. Therefore, building connections on the phone is critical.

The telephone, although far from being a new technology, still presents challenges and the potential for miscommunication. Phone calls are solely oral-verbal and auditory by nature. So, one of the greatest hurdles is the limited ability to send and receive nonverbal messages, potentiating misunderstandings. During telephone conversations, it is difficult to determine when our spoken communication is unclear. Without visual cues – facial expressions, gestures, body positioning, and postures – to guide or alert us, we miss chances to clarify what we mean.

So, to enhance understanding, enunciate words and keep verbal statements short, simple, and succinct. Also pause longer for responses, and do not be shy about requesting clarification. Be conscious of and use vocal nonverbal cues detected over the telephone, such as voice volume, tone, rate of speech, and pacing. Before picking up the telephone: take a breath, focus, and slow down; then, prepare to use a warm voice to welcome the caller to the veterinary practice. Finally, implement the three opening communication skills – preparation, introduction, and agenda-setting – for exemplary telephone etiquette (Box 3.3).

Box 3.3   Using Opening-the-Interaction Communication Skills on the Telephone

Preparation: First, take a deep breath to put aside all other distractions and reset.

Introduction: *Hello, this is Jesse,* [make introduction to the client] *the client service coordinator at <name> Animal Hospital.* [clarify your role] *Thanks for calling.* [demonstrate interest] *How can I help you?* [reason(s) for visit]

Agenda Setting: *Hello, Mr. Dolohov. So, you'd like to schedule an appointment for Francis with Dr. Morrison because he's **losing weight**.* [summarize client's agenda] *What other concerns would you like to discuss with Dr. Morrison?* [concerns]

*Okay. So, in addition to Francis's **weight loss**, I put in the appointment notes that you'd like to take a **different approach**.* [summarize client's agenda] *What else are you hoping we can do for Francis during your visit?* [expectations]

*Sounds like you'd like Dr. Morrison to determine the **cause of the weight loss** so that you can get Francis back on track.* [summarize client's agenda]

We have an opening tomorrow at 2:00 p.m. Would that work for you and Francis? How else can I help you today? [check]

*You're very welcome. We're looking forward to seeing you and Francis tomorrow, Tuesday, May 28, at 2 p.m., to sort out Francis's **weight loss problem**. If you have concerns with Francis before then, please give me a call back.*

Opening Team Interactions

As with client interactions, be intentional about opening conversations with colleagues. Greet colleagues at the start of the day, ask how they are doing, and slow down and pay attention to their responses. Kick off staff meetings with a friendly opening and expressions of gratitude. Extend a hand and provide a warm welcome to visitors to the practice. All of these help colleagues feel like valued team members, allow the day or meeting to get off to a productive start, and establish a collaborative team culture (Sidebar 3.5).

Sidebar 3.5   Team Outcomes of an Effective Opening

Foster satisfaction
Support positive culture
Enhance efficiency
Promote retention
Provide structure
Improve recruitment

Follow the same skills outlined in "Opening Client Interactions" (preparation, introduction, and agenda-setting) to open interactions with colleagues, whether individual interactions or group meetings. Prepare for meetings with colleagues: reflect on the agenda ahead of time; review past notes, email exchanges, or lists of topics; and anticipate possible issues or questions. If there is no time to prepare between meetings, be transparent and ask colleague(s) for a briefing. *I've been tracking the email exchanges. Would you mind starting with summarizing the key concerns?*

Ensure that everyone in attendance is acquainted, and introduce new colleagues. Take a minute to go around the table and ask *How are you doing?* Or conduct a pulse check, asking *On a scale from 1 to 5, where 1 is your worst day ever and 5 is the best, what is your rating, and why?* Or ask, *What adjective would you use to describe your day, and why?* This informal pulse check provides a quick assessment of the team and a sense of a starting point, with group acknowledgment of reasons for celebration or stressors, distractions, or challenges that could otherwise derail the meeting. Checking in assesses the team's capabilities, preparedness, and readiness to accomplish the meeting tasks.

Then establish a mutually agreed-on agenda. First, review the proposed meeting agenda. Next, request additional items from the team; then, as a group, prioritize what to achieve during the session. The final shared agenda highlights the order of topics to be addressed and provides direction and mile markers for how the meeting will proceed.

Routine Team Scenario

Set the Scene: Today the practice is hosting Jill Fritz, a registered veterinary technician, for a day-long onsite interview. The first meeting is with Mario, the practice manager, Sharma, the leader of the client service team, and Andrea, the lead veterinary technician.

Preparation: The interview team creates an itinerary for Jill's visit and invites and informs all the key players to meet with Jill during the day.

Introductions:

MARIO: *Hi, Jill. I'm Mario, the practice manager and I use he/him pronouns.* [make introduction to colleague and clarify your role] *Thanks for spending the day with us. We're looking forward to getting to know you.* [demonstrate interest] *Let me ask Sharma and Andrea to introduce themselves.*

SHARMA: *Hi, Jill. It's great to meet you! I'm Sharma, I supervise the client service coordinators, and I use they/them pronouns.* [make introduction to colleague and clarify your role]

ANDREA: *I'm Andrea, the lead technician, I use she/her pronouns,* [make introduction to colleague and clarify your role] *and we'll spend a good part of the day together.* [demonstrate interest]

Agenda-Setting:

MARIO: *We have a full itinerary for you today, including meetings with practice team members this morning and time allotted for a working interview this afternoon.* [practice team's agenda] *We'd also like to know what you'd like to get out of your interview visit today.* [goals]

MARIO: *What else are you hoping to learn about our practice?* [expectations]

MARIO: *That's not a problem. We can find time to give you a demonstration of our **practice management and electronic medical record systems.** Andrea can show you our **anesthesia monitoring equipment,** and I'll be sure to ask the practice owner, Dr. Callahan, to go over **team scheduling** with you.* [summarize colleague's agenda] *What else is on your list?* [check]

Challenging Team Scenario

Set the Scene: During Jill's working interview, Lindsey, one of the veterinary technicians, comes into the treatment room to schedule Francis, the rabbit, for an oral examination. Dr. Hernandez is concerned that Francis may have a tooth abscess and would like the procedure scheduled as soon as possible. Andrea, the lead veterinary technician, is managing the treatment room schedule this afternoon.

Preparation: As Lindsey walks into the treatment room, she conducts a quick assessment, sees that Andrea's hands are full, and considers how to present her request.

Introductions:

LINDSEY: *Hi, Andrea. What's the schedule looking like for this afternoon?*

ANDREA: *Unfortunately, we're fully booked. But I'm glad to see you, Lindsey, because I'd like to introduce you to Jill. She's doing her working interview this afternoon.* [make introduction to colleague and clarify your role]

LINDSEY: *Nice to meet you, Jill. I'm Lindsey. I'm one of the veterinary technicians here and I use she/her pronouns.* [make introduction to colleague and clarify your role] *I'll be available later for anything you'd like to ask me or talk to me about.* [demonstrate interest]

Agenda-setting:

LINDSEY: *So, Andrea, Dr. Hernandez is really concerned about Francis, as he's lost a lot of weight, and he would like to fit him in as soon as possible.* [summarize Dr. Hernandez's agenda] *What are the possibilities of squeezing him in this afternoon?* [priorities]

ANDREA: *There's not much wiggle room in today's schedule.* [colleague's agenda]

LINDSEY: *I saw on the board that several patients need radiographs.* [colleague's agenda] *What if I were to get the radiographs done after my appointments? Would that help to free up a time slot for Francis?* [negotiate a mutual agenda]

ANDREA: *That just might work! While you're taking the radiographs, I can set up for Francis, and then we can both assist Dr. Hernandez with Francis's oral examination.* [summarize the mutually agreed-on agenda] *It'll also give me a few minutes to answer any questions Jill may have. How does that sound?* [check]

Put the Opening Skills into Practice

Do-It-Yourself Exercises

Exercise 3.1   Skill Spot – Introduction

Review the following examples of introductions for an appointment that is running late. Identify what items are **missing** from the introduction (Sidebar 3.3). The answer key is posted at the end of the chapter.

1. *Hi, Mr. Dolohov. I'm Dr. Hernandez, one of the veterinarians here at <Veterinary Practice>. Hello there, Francis! How is Francis doing?*

2. *Hi, Mr. Dolohov. Sorry to keep you waiting. I'm Vanessa and I use she/her pronouns. How would you prefer to be addressed? It sounds like you are concerned about Francis.*

3. *Hi, Mr. Dolohov. I'm Dr. Hernandez. You can call me Vanessa and I use she/her pronouns. I am one of the veterinarians here at <Veterinary Practice>. This must be Francis; he's cute! I appreciate your waiting, and I'm sorry that I am running behind.*

Exercise 3.2 Skill Spot – Agenda-Setting

Review the following examples of agenda-setting. Identify which items are **missing** from the agenda-setting steps (Sidebar 3.4). See the end of the chapter for the answer key.

1. *What brings you and Francis in today? So, you are concerned that Francis is losing weight, no matter what we try.*

2. *What would you like to discuss in today's visit? So, Francis continues to lose weight no matter what we've tried so far. I would also like to ask about his eating habits and diet and then identify next steps.*

3. *What other concerns do you have for today's visit? What are you hoping we can do for Francis? I'd like to learn more about his eating habits and diet, and then we can figure out how to get to the bottom of this. What else would you like to discuss?*

Exercise 3.3 Next Steps for Success

Trying on a new communication approach is awkward. It takes effort to become automatic and authentic. Be gentle and kind. At the same time, stretch to move through the awkward phase to feel more comfortable, confident, and competent.

1. Work through the first two opening communication skills by focusing on one at a time. Start with preparation, and then introduction and consciously practice the skills.

2. When you are ready, identify a coaching partner in the practice. Inform them of the goals you set for the preparation or introduction skills, invite them to observe the interaction at a mutually convenient time, and request balanced, descriptive, detailed feedback about the selected skill.

3. Once you are confident, repeat the cycle by honing in on the other opening communication skill. Practice, then request feedback from a colleague, and continue conducting self-assessments until you achieve competence.

Exercise 3.4 Track Agenda-Setting Results

Next, focus on the third opening skill: agenda-setting. Depending on your practice role, self-reflect on a client or colleague conversation. For the next month, during clinical appointments or colleague interactions, conduct an experiment – individually, with a peer coach, or as a team – to focus on agenda-setting with clients or colleagues (Sidebar 3.4). Use these instructions as a guide to log the outcomes:

1. After each interaction, write down all of your client's or colleague's agenda items revealed and tally them up.

2. Label each as:
   a. Reason(s) for the visit/meeting
   b. Client or colleague concerns
   c. Goals, priorities, or expectations

3. Note whether a client or colleague concern was raised at the end of the visit.

4. Write down the visit or meeting length.

5. At the end of the month, review the notes, and identify trends over time (e.g. number of concerns identified, number of issues raised at the end, and overall length of appointments/ meetings). See what happens with more proficiency with agenda-setting over time.

Engage-the-Entire-Team Exercise

Exercise 3.5   Role-Play: The Hand-Off
The purpose of this exercise is to practice handing off the client's agenda between team members, as naturally occurs within the cycle of each appointment. The client reveals their initial agenda to the client service coordinator or representative over the phone, the veterinary technician clarifies the agenda in person with the client and shares the agenda with the veterinarian, and the veterinarian confirms with the client if the agenda is accurate (Box 3.2). New agenda items may be revealed during each team member interaction.

Participants: Conduct this exercise in a small group of four team members, ideally a client service coordinator or representative, two veterinary technicians, and a veterinarian.

1. Prepare one individual to role-play a **client**:
   a. Ask if a veterinary technician or client service coordinator or representative would be willing to play the role of a client.
   b. To identify a case scenario, ask them to consider a time when they brought their own animal to the veterinary clinic or to recall a recent client visit and that client's agenda.
   c. To get into their role, let them take a minute to reflect on an agenda for the visit (e.g. reason(s), concerns, goals, priorities, and expectations)
   d. Request that they share agenda items over time as questions are asked, revealing the easier reasons initially and then more concerning items later. Clients often disclose sensitive topics only after they feel rapport and comfort with a veterinary team member.

2. **Client service coordinator or representative** (over the phone) or **veterinary technician** (in person):
   a. Obtain the client's agenda, including:
      i. Reason(s) for the visit – *What brings you and <animal's name> in today?*
      ii. Client concerns for the pet – *What concerns would you like to discuss?*
      iii. Goals, priorities, and expectations – *What are your goals for today's visit?*
   b. Summarize the agenda back to the client – *So, you and <animal's name> are scheduled for x, y, and z.*
   c. Check – *What else can I help you with today?*

3. **Veterinary technician**:
   a. Review the appointment notes or obtain the client's agenda from the client service coordinator or representative (as outlined earlier).

b. Summarize the agenda to the client – *I read in the appointment notes that you are concerned about x, y, and z.*

c. Check – *What else would you like to discuss with Dr. <name> today?*

d. Present the case and summarize the agenda to the veterinarian – *<Client name> and <animal name> are here today for x, y, and z; their greatest concerns are . . ., the biggest issue is . . ., and the main goal for today's visit is . . .*

4. **Veterinarian**:

a. Summarize the agenda back to the client – *<Veterinary technician's name> shared with me that you are here today for x, y, and z, and your priority is to . . .*

b. Check with the client – *What else would you like to talk about today?*

5. Repeat this exercise multiple times, taking turns role-playing the client until each team member feels confident and competent in eliciting, summarizing, and checking in on the client's agenda.

Take It Away

1. **Prepare** mentally before the appointment or meeting to be present and give your full attention to the client, patient, or colleague.

2. Open your client interaction or team meeting with a strong **introduction**, including exchange of names, how they'd like to be addressed, and clarifying the roles of all those in attendance; demonstrate interest; and acknowledge any immediate concerns up front.

3. **Fully elicit your client's or colleague's agenda** early on to identify reason(s) for the interaction or meeting; obtain their list of concerns; and request goals, expectations, and priorities. Summarize what you heard, and check for any remaining items. Then introduce your agenda items, and meld your agenda with that of your client or colleague. Summarize again the mutually agreed-on agenda for moving forward, and check to be sure it is right.

Answer Key

Exercise 3.1   Skill Spot – Introduction

1. *Hi, Mr. Dolohov. I'm Dr. Hernandez,* [make introduction to the client] *one of the veterinarians here at <Veterinary Practice>.* [clarify your role] *Hello there, Francis!* [make introduction to the pet] *How is Francis doing?* [demonstrate interest]

   What is missing?
   a. Invite client to introduce themselves and their pet
   b. Address immediate concern(s) that the schedule is running behind.

2. *Hi, Mr. Dolohov. Sorry to keep you waiting.* [address immediate concern(s)] *I'm Vanessa and I use she/her pronouns.* [make introduction to the client] *How would you prefer to be*

addressed? [invite client to introduce themselves] *It sounds like you are concerned about Francis.* [demonstrate interest]

What is missing?
   a. Clarify your role
   b. Make introduction to the pet

3. *Hi, Mr. Dolohov. I'm Dr. Hernandez. You can call me Vanessa and I use she/her pronouns.* [make introduction to the client] *I am one of the veterinarians here at <Veterinary Practice>.* [clarify your role] *This must be Francis* [make introduction to the pet]; *he's cute!* [demonstrate interest] *I appreciate your waiting, and I'm sorry that I am running behind.* [address immediate concern(s)]

    What is missing?
       a. Invite client to introduce themselves and their pet.
       b. Demonstrate interest in Mr. Dolohov.

To close this exercise, we provide an example of a **complete introduction**, including all five steps for reference:

Hi Mr. Dolohov. I'm Dr. Hernandez. You can call me Vanessa and I use she/her pronouns. [make introduction to the client] *I am one of the veterinarians here at <Veterinary Practice>.* [clarify your role] *How would you prefer to be addressed?* [invite client to introduce themselves] *I am sorry that we've kept you waiting and that Dr. Morrison is unavailable.* [address immediate concern(s)] *Oh, this is Francis* [introduction to pet] *– he's a handsome fella!* [demonstrate interest] *It's nice to meet you both; Dr. Morrison filled me in on what's been going on with Francis.* [demonstrate interest]

Exercise 3.2   Skill Spot – Agenda-Setting

1. *What brings you and Francis in today?* [reason(s) for visit] *So, you are concerned that Francis is losing weight, no matter what we try.* [summarize client's agenda]

    What is missing?
       a. Elicit client's concerns, goals, expectations, and priorities
       b. Check for remaining items
       c. Offer veterinary professional's agenda
       d. Negotiate a mutual agenda
       e. Summarize the mutually agreed-on agenda

2. *What would you like to discuss in today's visit?* [reason(s) for visit] *So, Francis continues to lose weight no matter what we've tried so far.* [summarize client's agenda] *I would also like to ask about his eating habits and diet and then identify next steps.* [offer veterinary professional's agenda]

    What is missing?
       a. Elicit client's concerns, goals, expectations, and priorities
       b. Check for remaining items

    c. Negotiate a mutual agenda

    d. Summarize the mutually agreed-on agenda

3. *What other concerns do you have for today's visit?* [concerns] *What are you hoping we can do for Francis?* [expectations] *I'd like to learn more about his eating habits and diet, and then we can figure out how to get to the bottom of this.* [offer veterinary professional's agenda] *What else would you like to discuss?* [check]

    What is missing?

        a. Elicit the reason(s) for the visit, goals, and priorities

        b. Summarize the client's agenda

        c. Negotiate a mutual agenda

        d. Summarize the mutually agreed-on agenda

To close this exercise, we provide an example of **complete agenda-setting,** including all six steps for reference:

What brings you and Francis in today? [reason(s) for visit]
What concerns you about Francis? [concerns]
What would make this a satisfying visit for you and Francis? [goals]
What are you hoping we can do for Francis? [expectations]
What is most important to you? [priorities]

I hear that we need to address Francis's **continued weight loss** *and* **lack of response to treatment** *and come up with a* **new plan**. [summarize client's agenda] *What else is on your mind for today's visit?* [check]

I'd like to learn more about Francis's **eating habits** *and* **diet**. [offer veterinary professional's agenda] *Would it be all right if I added that to our list?* After our discussion, w*ould you be comfortable leaving Francis with us this afternoon, so we can sedate him and perform a complete examination of his mouth?* [negotiate a mutual agenda]

What's on our plate today is to discuss Francis's **weight loss**, *review his* **dietary habits**, *sedated* **examination of his mouth**, *and then come up with a* **plan** *to get him back on track.* [summarize mutually agreed-on agenda] *What have I missed?* [check]

References

Beckman, H.B. and Frankel, R.M. (1984). The effect of physician behavior on the collection of patient data. *Ann. Intern. Med.* 101 (5): 692–696. https://doi.org/10.7326/0003-4819-101-5-692.

Dysart, L.M.A., Coe, J.B., and Adams, C.L. (2011). Analysis of solicitation of client concerns in companion animal practice. *J. Am. Vet. Med. Assoc.* 238 (12): 1609–1615. https://doi.org/10.2460/javma.238.12.1609.

Hunter, L. and Shaw, J.R. (2011). *The Art of Initiation.* Exceptional Veterinary Team. May/June: 5–8.

4

Information-Gathering

Abstract

A complete and accurate history serves as the foundation on which diagnostic and treatment planning, problem-solving, and solution-generating rely. Information-gathering in veterinary practice is a team sport, involving multiple steps and colleagues. In this chapter, we discuss the role of information-gathering not only to flesh out the medical details but also to understand the client, the patient, and their environmental context. We discuss how to elicit the client's or our colleague's novel perspective. Taking a less interrogative and more conversational approach initially may feel as though it is slowing the process; however, with the whole clinical picture and clear client or colleague viewpoints identified up front, the interaction proceeds more rapidly in the long run. We explore five communication skills for gathering information with clients and colleagues: open-ended inquiry, closed-ended inquiry, pause, minimal encouragers, and reflective listening.

SELF-ASSESSMENT QUESTIONS

1. How much do I learn up front about my patient, client, and their environment, or my colleague's situation, perspective, and their environment?
2. What is my information-gathering style: interrogation or conversation?
3. How extensive is my picture of my patient's, client's, or colleague's story?

Introduction

A complete and accurate history serves as the foundation on which diagnostic and treatment planning, problem-solving, and solution-generating rely. Traditionally, information-gathering focused on the animal patient and making the diagnosis. Now, we gather information not only to flesh out the medical details but also to understand the client, the patient, and their environmental context. Exploring where the client is coming from and conducting an environmental assessment identifies potential risk factors and barriers to client adherence.

Clients are experts on the animals they live with: they know about their environment and household; their time and financial resources; and their pet's temperament, lifestyle, and interactions. The client's observations of their pet are critical, as their impressions "speak" for the patient's clinical signs. All of these are invaluable for arriving at an accurate diagnosis and

Developing Communication Skills for Veterinary Practice, First Edition. Jane R. Shaw and Jason B. Coe.
© 2024 John Wiley & Sons, Inc. Published 2024 by John Wiley & Sons, Inc.

proposing to the client a medically sound, customized, and practical treatment plan (Sidebar 4.1 and Research Spotlight 4.1).

Sidebar 4.1   Clinical Outcomes of Effective Information-Gathering

Improve efficiency
Enhance client satisfaction
Promote diagnostic accuracy
Increase client adherence to recommendations

Research Spotlight 4.1

Time Spent Gathering Information

In a detailed analysis of 300 video recordings of veterinarian-client-patient interactions (Shaw et al. 2004), 10% of the appointment was spent information-gathering. Given the value of a full history in diagnosing the patient and meeting client expectations, we may be rushing through information-gathering. Eliciting the patient's biomedical data, the client's perspective, and a thorough environmental scan likely requires a shift from 10% to at least 30% of time spent information-gathering. Front-end loading of the history results in a more efficient, targeted, and customized diagnostic and treatment planning process later in the appointment. These results emphasize the importance of taking time to get the full clinical picture before launching into formulating a plan.

When we gather a history, we walk a tightrope between collecting relevant patient biomedical data thoroughly and efficiently while attending to the client's expectations, needs, and concerns and getting a clear picture of the setting. As each client is unique, we often need to ask questions about their beliefs, opinions, values, and priorities. Doing so ensures that we keep an open mind, do not make assumptions, and check our biases, leaving judgments at the door. The same is true when working with colleagues to ensure that we do not jump to conclusions prematurely. We first gain an appreciation for what it is like to walk in our client's or colleague's shoes.

Information-gathering in veterinary practice is a team sport. It starts with what is shared with the client service coordinator or representative over the phone or on the initial presentation to the reception desk. Next, the veterinary technician often obtains the foundation of the history. Then the veterinarian digs deeper, clarifying details and striving to gain a robust picture of what is going on with the patient and for the client. Because the information-gathering task is shared, continuity of communication between team members is essential to ensure that the history passed on is correct and thorough.

Every day, hour, and minute, we feel the time crunch at work. So, it is understandable that we often rush through information-gathering using an interrogative approach. It is common to pose yes/no questions designed to focus on the vital information we believe will solve the clinical case as quickly as possible. This also happens in team interactions: we want to quickly find the problem, fix it, and move on.

Yet this approach jeopardizes diagnostic accuracy and client or colleague relationship-building by missing key pieces of information. We leap to conclusions before obtaining a clear and comprehensive understanding of the problem. Taking a less interrogative and more conversational approach initially may feel as though it slows the process; however, with the whole clinical picture and clear client or colleague viewpoints identified up front, the interaction proceeds more rapidly in the long run.

In his 2007 book *How Doctors Think*, Jerome Groopman recounts one patient tale after another of how doctors missed key historical details and misdiagnosed their patients. When subsequent doctors went back to conduct a complete and thorough history, the lost puzzle pieces were identified, and they were able to make accurate diagnoses and initiate the correct treatments. The most disheartening aspects were the number of doctor visits, the batteries of unnecessary diagnostic tests, and the long periods of patient suffering before answers were found. Lesson learned: before requesting bloodwork, urinalysis, radiograph, ultrasound, endoscopy, CT scan, or MRI, consider pulling up a chair and fully exploring the patient, client, and environmental history with full attention.

In this chapter, we discuss how to explore the patient's biomedical information or the team's challenge in a way that appreciates the client's or our colleague's novel perspective. Multiple lists provide example questions to gather patient, client, and environment data or colleague's situation, perspective, and environment data and gain a comprehensive picture. Pick and choose questions based on what is already known from prior client or colleague interactions and the medical record and what requires more insight. Let the reasoning process guide the identification of the most appropriate questions.

Further, we explore five communication skills for gathering information with clients and colleagues: open-ended inquiry, closed-ended inquiry, pause, minimal encouragers, and reflective listening (Sidebar 4.2). We provide examples in three locations: in the examination room, interacting with Ms. Srinivasan and her dog, Buddy; in a team meeting led by Dalia, the practice manager; and in a meeting between Dalia and Stacey, a veterinary technician, regarding roles and responsibilities.

Sidebar 4.2   Five Communication Skills for Information-Gathering

Open-ended inquiry
Closed-ended inquiry
Pause
Minimal encouragers
Reflective listening

Set the Scene

Client Scenario

Ms. Srinivasan presents with Buddy, a six-year-old male-castrated Labrador retriever, to see Dr. Patel for limping. On presentation, Buddy is toe-touching lame on his right-hind limb.

Team Scenarios

Dalia is a practice manager at a busy, multi-doctor practice with dozens of employees. One of her responsibilities is scheduling shifts. She recently released the new team schedule, which was received with complaints and dissatisfaction. She calls a team meeting to hear employee concerns.

Afterward, Dalia requests an individual meeting with Stacey, one of the veterinary technicians, to review roles and responsibilities. Dalia overheard a conversation in which Stacey seemed to be struggling to take a more team-oriented approach to her job.

Stepping into Dr. Patel's and Dalia's shoes, self-reflect on:

1. How would I gather a complete understanding of Buddy's lameness and overall health, Ms. Srinivasan's perspective, and their surrounding environment?
2. How would I fully elicit my colleagues' scheduling concerns?
3. How would I approach Stacey with my concern about her performance?

Gather Patient, Client, and Environment Information

Attend to the Process of Information-Gathering with Clients

The process, or the **how**, of information-gathering is using key communication skills to gather biomedical data, client perspective, and environmental information. One self-assessment question when conducting a history is, **Who is doing the most talking?** During information-gathering, it is expected that clients will do most of the talking, sharing details about their situation and their astute observations of their pet. When veterinary professionals interrogate clients to obtain a history, we do all the work and leave little room for the client to speak. When information-gathering is conversational, the workload is shared. It takes the burden off the veterinary professional, puts the storytelling on the client, and often reveals details we may not even considered asking about.

A critical difference between the two approaches (i.e. interrogation vs. conversation) is our capacity to truly listen to our client. While interrogating, we are often in our own heads, thinking of the next question rather than being attentive and listening to the client's responses. In the conversational mode, we focus on what the client is saying, picking up key verbal and nonverbal cues and then exploring them more deeply. If we listen closely, the client's responses naturally lead us to the next question to be posed.

Information-gathering involves three main tasks: asking questions, listening to responses, and processing information (Box 4.1). The mindful attention paid to these steps determines the quality of the data gathered, so be aware of the phrasing of questions, be present in the moment, listen carefully to the client, and pause longer than is usually comfortable to give the client space to share.

Box 4.1   The "How" of Client Information-Gathering

1. **Ask questions:**
   a. Start with broad, open-ended inquiry then focused open-ended inquiry.
   b. Follow up with specific, closed-ended inquiry to clarify details.

2. **Listen to the responses:**
   a. Pause for at least three seconds of silence after asking each question, being mindful not to interrupt the other person.
   b. Listen attentively, using minimal encouragers.
   c. Demonstrate active listening through attentive nonverbal cues (e.g. eye contact, nodding, sitting forward, leaning in, and turning toward the client).

3. **Process the information:**

    a. Pause to self-reflect and ask yourself:

        i. *What have I learned so far?*

        ii. *What do I need to know more about?*

        iii. *What am I still curious about?*

        iv. *What areas need further clarification?*

    b. Use reflective techniques to show you are listening and to confirm, correct, or clarify what the client said.

    c. Summarize to pull together all the key details you heard, to benefit you and the other person.

Key Communication Skills for Information-Gathering

Open-Ended Inquiry

Definition
Includes both questions and statements that draw out a broad response from clients by inviting them to tell a story. Open-ended inquiry encourages our clients to share events in their own words; provide detailed accounts of their concerns or frustrations; describe problems, clinical signs, context, and history; and offer solutions.

Technique
Open-ended inquiry begins with stems that invite elaboration (Sidebar 4.3).

Sidebar 4.3 Open-Ended Inquiry Stems

What . . .
How . . .
Tell me . . .
Walk me through . . .
Describe for me . . .
Explain to me . . .
Elaborate on . . .
Share with me . . .
Help me understand . . .
Paint a picture of . . .

There are several challenges to using open-ended inquiry: phrasing what, how, and why questions, compound questions, and providing multiple choice questions. It is important to note that while *how* and *what* are commonly considered stems for generating open-ended inquiries, they also serve as stems for closed-ended questions. *What* and *how* questions phrased broadly at the mouth of the funnel are open-ended. As we move down the funnel, *what* and *how* questions become more focused and closed. Therefore, when using *what* and *how* questions that are intended to be open-ended, be careful that the question is truly inviting and nonleading (Research Spotlight 4.2).

Research Spotlight 4.2

Impact of Open-Ended Inquiries

In a study of veterinarians' conversations with clients about their pet's nutrition, it was found that *what*-prefaced questions used to explore the pet's diet (e.g. *What kind of food is he eating?*) were treated by both veterinarians and clients as closed-ended. This resulted in clients responding with limited information, predominantly brand-related information about their pet's commercial diet (MacMartin et al. 2015).

In a follow-up study examining the effects of three different diet-history questions, client responses differed when asked this broad, open-ended inquiry: *Tell me everything he eats throughout a day, starting first thing in the morning right through to the end of the day* compared to the *what*-prefaced diet-history question. The study found that the more open-ended form of inquiry elicited almost three times the total number of diet-related items (Coe et al. 2020). This finding reinforces that the broader the open-ended inquiry, the more information is revealed.

In addition, attempt to avoid questions that begin with *why*. Asking *why* questions puts people on the defensive or feel intimidating because a *why* question sounds like it requires justification. The more we practice phrasing open-ended inquiry, the more skilled we become. That said, a solid default is *Tell me more.*

Examples

> Ms. Srinivasan, **tell me** what is going on with Buddy. [open-ended inquiry]
> **Describe for me** the progression of Buddy's lameness. [focused open-ended inquiry]
> **What** seems to make his lameness worse? [focused open-ended inquiry]
> **What** are you giving Buddy for his lameness? [focused open-ended inquiry]

In our urgency to get the answers, we tend to pose more than one open-ended inquiry or ask about multiple topics at the same time (i.e. compound questions). It is difficult for clients to track more than one subject, and they often only answer one of the questions posed. Ask one open-ended inquiry at a time and pause to gather a more complete picture.

A final difficulty is qualifying our open-ended inquiry with a list of potential options (i.e. a multiple choice question). In our rush to learn more, we fill in the blank and list several responses for the client. The consequence is closing down our open-ended inquiry. Stick with your open-ended inquiry, take a pause, and wait for the client to respond.

Open-ended inquiry is a foundational skill and will be revisited multiple times throughout this book. It was already introduced as a critical tool for eliciting the client's full agenda. Coming up, it is an integral instrument to check with the client after an internal or end summary to see if something was missed, during chunk-and-check to assess the client's understanding, and as a final check to see if everything was addressed.

Use the Inquiry Funnel

When gathering information, we recommend using the inquiry funnel technique. Funnelling starts with general, catchall inquiries and then focused inquiries and collimates down with narrow, closed-ended questions. Begin with broad, open-ended inquiries to paint a picture of the problem(s), followed by more focused open-ended inquiries to explore areas for further

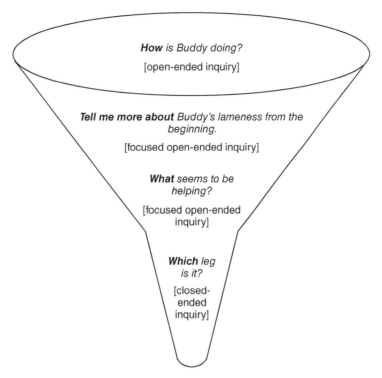

Figure 4.1 The inquiry funnel.

information, and end with fine-tuned, specific, direct questions that clarify the details and complete the picture. Figure 4.1 depicts a funnel script with a broad, open-ended inquiry at the funnel's opening, working down the funnel with more focused open-ended inquiries, and ending with a specific closed-ended question to complete the picture of Buddy's lameness at the funnel's outlet.

Information-gathering is much like putting together a complex jigsaw puzzle. When the client and patient come in, all the puzzle pieces lie haphazardly on the exam room table. The veterinary professional's role is to put the puzzle together and come up with a diagnosis and recommend a treatment plan. To do so, use an open-ended inquiry to grab a handful of puzzle pieces and put quadrants of the puzzle together, or ask a closed question to reach for one puzzle piece at a time. We quickly see that putting the puzzle together is more efficient using open-ended inquiry. Pose closed-ended inquiries to place the final pieces and complete the puzzle.

Traditionally, information-gathering was taught and modeled using closed-ended inquiries. Many veterinary professionals identify with these inquiries: *Any vomiting? Any diarrhea? Any coughing? Any sneezing? Any lameness? Any lumps or bumps?* This upside-down funnel approach is much like the "Twenty Questions" guessing game. The conversation rhythm is interrogative as the veterinary professional rapidly shoots closed-ended inquiries, hoping to make an accurate diagnosis (Research Spotlight 4.3).

The client's responses to closed-ended inquiries offer critical pieces of biomedical information. And starting more broadly (e.g. *Describe Buddy's lameness over the past week*), followed by a closed-ended inquiry when characteristics are left out by the client (e.g. *Does it get worse after his walk?*), provides an even fuller picture and reduces the risk of a client inadvertently leaving out an important piece of information. After most of the story is learned from open-ended inquiry, closed-ended inquiries catch key details that remain and provide an opportunity for clarification.

Research Spotlight 4.3

The Funnel Is Upside-Down

Detailed quantitative analysis of video recordings of 300 veterinarian-client interactions revealed that, on average, veterinarians asked 13 closed-ended inquiries per appointment versus 2 open-ended inquiries. In 25% of the appointments, veterinarians did not pose any open-ended inquiries (Shaw et al. 2004). Closed-ended inquiry limits exploration, impacting the quality of data gathering and, subsequently, the formulation of an accurate diagnosis. This contrasts with the upright funnel of using predominantly open-ended inquiry and then asking clarifying closed-ended inquiries to fill in the gaps or identify missing data. These findings highlight that there are opportunities for veterinary professionals to use more open-ended inquiry to gather a more refined and robust history.

Closed-Ended Inquiry

Definition

Results in specific, simple, and often one-word client responses. Closed-ended questioning best serves as a clean-up technique to fill in remaining information gaps. Following the use of broader open-ended inquiry, the purpose of using closed-ended inquiry is to gather final details to complete the client's story, leaving no stone unturned. Asking permission is a special form of closed-ended inquiry presented in Chapter 5. Asking permission uses sensitive, gentle, and respectful phrasing (*Shall we, Is it alright if, or Would it be okay if*) that invites a client to accept or decline the opportunity to share.

Technique

Closed-ended questions are often phrased with stems requesting specificity and prompt a yes/no or one-word answer (Sidebar 4.4).

> **Sidebar 4.4   Closed-ended Inquiry Stems**
>
> *When . . .*
> *Where . . .*
> *Which . . .*
> *Are/Is . . .*
> *Do/Does . . .*
> *Have/has . . .*
> *Can/could . . .*
> *Will/would . . .*

Examples

> **Has** *Buddy been vomiting?*
> **Has** *he been coughing?*
> **Is** *he in discomfort?*
> **Have** *you tried anything?*
> **Are** *you limiting his exercise?*

Pause

Definition
Silence accompanied by nonverbal presence – maintaining eye contact, nodding, facing and sitting with the client, leaning in, and displaying interested facial expressions and calm gestures – invites elaboration and allows the client to tell their full story and signals that we are here to listen.

Technique
Pause entails using silence for emphasis, reflection or processing (Sidebar 4.5).

Sidebar 4.5   Pause Strategies

Count for three (or more) seconds
Take several deep breaths
Listen to the ambient noises in the room
Be present to and aware of our own thoughts
Reflect on what we heard or learned so far

Example
> *Ms. Srinivasan, tell me more. <Pause: one, one thousand; two, one thousand; three, one thousand>*

Avoid Interruptions

Equally important to how we pose questions is our ability to pause and patiently wait for the client to answer. A well-worded open-ended inquiry requires thought to answer. The client needs time to reflect on where and how to begin and what information to present and, at the same time, recall the key details. If it is worth asking about, it is worth patiently waiting for the client's response.

When we restrain ourselves from interrupting, the client finishes their thought, elaborates on what they said, and closes their story. If the client is interrupted before concluding, they often do not complete their response, leaving holes or omitting data that may be critical to making an accurate diagnosis. It is the veterinary professional's responsibility to minimize interruptions and hold a "pause" in the dialogue (Research Spotlight 4.4).

Research Spotlight 4.4

Consequences of Interruptions

In a study investigating the solicitation of client concerns, veterinarians interrupted clients on average 15.3 seconds into their statement, thereby cutting off the expression of their whole story or list. In 28% of appointments in which clients were interrupted, the client returned to their concerns and completed their thoughts. In the other 72% of appointments, clients did not return to their concerns, and the veterinarian potentially missed key information (Dysart et al. 2011). These findings highlight the need for veterinary professionals to be aware of interrupting clients to enhance the accuracy of data gathering.

Just as teachers and students are uncomfortable with silence in the classroom and business executives in the boardroom, so are veterinarians and clients in the examination room. If the veterinary professional creates a quiet space and waits long enough, eventually the client will speak, and they often share something important. The challenge is sitting out the awkward pause, much like the staring and blinking game we played as kids. Along with the kinds of questions asked, using a strategic pause is one of the best tools to elicit more information and encourage participation – and it requires no effort on our part: only patience and mindfulness.

Minimal Encouragers

Definition
Small phrases that invite the client to continue speaking.

Technique
Judicious use of minimal encouragers invites the client to share more (Sidebar 4.6). Beware, of overuse or too-frequent repetition, as these verbal encouragers can serve as interrupters or sound dismissive. Also watch the use of *okay*, which communicates "let's move on to the next thing" and creates a hurried or rushed atmosphere.

Sidebar 4.6   Minimal Encouragers

Go on . . .
Yes . . .
Hmm . . .
Um-hum . . .
Uh-huh . . .
I see . . .
Oh . . .
Wow . . .
Really . . .

Examples
Consider the following example:

> **VETERINARIAN:**   *How* did Buddy's lameness begin? [open-ended inquiry]
> **CLIENT:**   *It started on Saturday after he slipped and fell on the ice.*
> **VETERINARIAN:**   *Oh?* [minimal encourager]
> **CLIENT:**   *His right leg slid out from underneath him, and he fell on his right hip.*

Compare that interaction with this one:

> **VETERINARIAN:**   *How* did Buddy's lameness begin? [open-ended inquiry]
> **CLIENT:**   *It started on Saturday after he slipped and fell on the ice.*
> **VETERINARIAN:**   *Okay.*
> **CLIENT:**   *Mhmm*
> **VETERINARIAN:** *Alright.*

Reflective Listening

Definition
Lets clients know they were heard. Reflective listening is a multi-tool. It builds rapport, satisfaction, and trust when our clients feel listened to. As a data-gathering tool, it invites clients to add to, confirm, or correct information. It structures the conversation and is used to direct the client's attention to a specific talking point, go back to a concern, or request more information on a topic.

We introduce internal summary in Chapter 6; it is a tool used throughout the appointment for capturing information gathered, structuring the conversation, and clarifying the treatment plan. Like reflective listening, internal summary involves repeating back information to let the client know that they were heard and that we grasped all the key details. How the two skills differ is that reflective listening captures one piece of information, and summary lists multiple (i.e. more than two) pieces of data and pulls them all together.

Technique
Reflective listening stems let the client know that we were listening (Sidebar 4.7).

Sidebar 4.7   Reflective Listening Stems

So . . .
I heard you say . . .
You said that . . .
You shared that . . .
It sounds like . . .
It seems like . . .
You mentioned that . . .

Verifying understanding is accomplished through levels of reflection, from superficial echoing or paraphrasing to deep interpretation and internal summary.

Examples
Echoing repeats back the words the client used.

> ***It sounds like*** *it was an "on and off" lameness, and now it's a "daily" occurrence.* [echoing]

Paraphrasing is restating in our own words the content and/or feelings behind the client's message.

> ***So,*** *you're worried about the costs of the x-rays?* [paraphrasing]

Interpreting is listening for what is underneath the message based on what the client says verbally and what they exhibit nonverbally. This is the deepest level of listening as we try to identify and understand someone's underlying meaning.

> *In requesting a referral,* ***you*** *want to ensure that Buddy is in the most qualified hands and gets the best possible care.* [interpreting]

Internal summary is reflecting back all that you heard in a list format.

> ***I'd like to check to make sure I have all the puzzle pieces****. Buddy's lameness started after he slipped and fell. It was off and on initially and now occurs daily. You are concerned that it is getting worse.* [internal summary] ***What*** *would you like to add?* [open-ended inquiry]

Attend to the Content of Information-Gathering with Clients

The content, or **what**, of a complete history is made up of three components: patient, client, and environmental data (Figure 4.2 and Sidebar 4.8) (Kurtz et al. 2003). Use the five skills to paint a complete picture of the history.

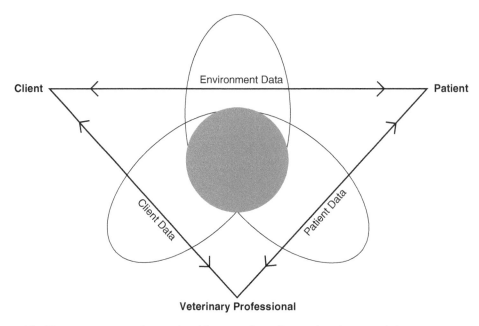

Figure 4.2 Three components of a complete history: patient, client and environmental data.

Sidebar 4.8   The "What" of Client Information-Gathering

1. **Patient data**

   a. **Current medical history**
      Sequence and progression of events
      Analysis of clinical signs
      Body-systems review

   b. **Past medical history**
      Role and function of the pet
      Past medical and surgical history
      Preventive medicine
      Nutrition
      Medication and supplement history
      Pet's temperament and behavior

2. **Client data or perspective**
   Acquisition of the pet
   Client's level of attachment to the pet
   Ideas and beliefs
   Thoughts and feelings
   Knowledge and experiences
   Information preferences
   Occupation
   Client lifestyle (schedule, routine, and financial resources)
   Pet caregivers' roles and responsibilities
   Impact of the pet's health on the animal's and client's lives

3. **Environmental data**

   Social interactions (human–human, human–animal, and animal–animal)

   Pet's activities of daily living (routine, feeding, exercise, sleeping habits, environmental enrichment, housing, and setting).

   Household lifestyle (schedule, routine, and travel)

   Recent life events (marriage/divorce, new additions, construction/renovations, recent move, and job stability)

Patient Data

The two components of patient data are the current and past medical history.

Current Medical History

The client's agenda items, especially the reason(s) for the visit and the client's concerns for the pet, outline the areas for investigation during information-gathering. For each, explore the sequence and progression of events, determine their duration or chronology, and conduct a full analysis of clinical signs and review of body systems:

Sequence and progression of events: A key objective of information-gathering is establishing the timeline, chronology, and duration of the illness (i.e. acute vs. chronic). Invite clients to tell their story of the events, from the beginning to this point in time, and describe how the pet's clinical signs progressed.

> **Tell me** *about Buddy's lameness from the beginning.* [focused open-ended inquiry]
> **Describe** *for me how the lameness has changed since you first noticed it.* [focused open-ended inquiry]

Analysis of clinical signs: Clinicians rely heavily on clients' descriptions, as clinical signs may not manifest in the examination room for observation. The picture that clients paint aids in refining the hypotheses or recognizing errors in the presumptive diagnoses. Open-ended inquiry encourages clients to tell a clear, detailed, and descriptive story of what they observed in their pet.

Using our knowledge of individual medical problems, we intelligently probe for additional information to formulate a problem list, develop rule-outs, and rank differential diagnoses. Start with open-ended inquiries, then focused open-ended inquiries and follow with closed-ended inquiries to narrowly target information associated with specific clinical problems. The questioning process aids in defining critical differentiations in clinical signs, such as vomiting versus regurgitation, syncope versus seizure, pollakiuria versus polyuria, and small versus large bowel diarrhea; or the body system origin, such as cardiac versus respiratory, cardiac versus neuromuscular, orthopedic versus neurologic, or medical versus behavioral problems.

> **Describe** *what his lameness looks like.* [focused open-ended inquiry]
> **What** *do you think makes him more painful?* [focused open-ended inquiry]

Body-systems review: This is a challenging part of the history because of the tendency to run down a checklist. To ensure that nothing is missed, rapid-fire, closed-ended inquiry often prevails. Although we are likely to uncover body-system abnormalities while exploring the client's agenda, it's also important to fully assess other organ systems. This critical step prevents us from getting tunnel vision. Strive for completeness through conversation versus interrogation to paint a comprehensive picture of the patient's health (Box 4.2).

Box 4.2   Conducting a Body-Systems Review Using Open-Ended Inquiry

There is a temptation to ask a checklist of closed-ended inquiries during the body-systems review (i.e. *Vomiting? Diarrhea? Coughing? Sneezing? Lumps/bumps? Lameness?*). However, the following open-ended checklist gathers a more complete patient history. Responses to these questions guide us in identifying body systems that may require a closer look during the physical examination.

Not all these systems need to be explored. Start with broad, general inquiries and then fill in the missing pieces with more focused, systems-based, open-ended inquiries. Reserve closed-ended inquiries to elicit or clarify details that may be left out.

General
> ***Describe*** *for me Buddy's overall health.*
> ***Tell me*** *about changes you've noticed in Buddy's health since his last visit.*
> ***What*** *else should I know about Buddy's health?*

Skin and haircoat
> ***Tell me*** *about Buddy's skin and hair coat.*
> ***Tell me*** *about any lumps or bumps you've found.*

Eyes, ears, nose, and throat
> ***Tell me*** *how you think Buddy sees/hears/smells <ask about one at a time>.*
> ***What*** *do you notice when Buddy is swallowing his food and water <ask about one at a time>?*

Respiratory
> ***Describe*** *for me Buddy's breathing on his walks.*
> ***How*** *would you characterize Buddy's breathing at rest/during sleep/while walking <ask about one at a time>?*

Cardiovascular
> ***Describe*** *Buddy's energy on his walks.*
> ***How would you describe*** *Buddy's endurance on walks?*

Gastrointestinal
> ***Characterize*** *Buddy's appetite for me.*
> ***Describe*** *Buddy's pooping habits.*
> ***What*** *changes have you noticed in Buddy's weight?*

Urinary
> ***Describe*** *Buddy's urinary habits.*
> ***Describe*** *Buddy's drinking habits.*

Reproductive
> ***Walk me*** *through Buddy's breeding history <if relevant>.*

Musculoskeletal/Nervous
> ***Tell me*** *about changes you've noticed in Buddy's physical activities.*
> ***How*** *does Buddy respond to stimuli around him?*
> ***How*** *is Buddy's balance?*

Past Medical History

The previous medical history provides a sturdy foundation and encompasses the role and function of the pet, past medical problems and surgical history, preventive medicine protocols, nutrition, medication and supplements, temperament, and behavior. Meeting new clients and patients warrants a full exploration of these topics, while for existing clients, only updates and documentation of any changes are required.

Role and function of the pet: Elicit the role the pet plays in the household and the pet's work duties (e.g. service, therapy, police, military, detection, search and rescue, herding), recreational activities (e.g. agility, flyball, disc, sledding, carting, canicross, tracking, dock jumping, Schutzhund, rally obedience, sheepdog tracking), and hobbies (e.g. walking, fetching, running, hiking, skiing, swimming).

> ***What*** *role does Buddy play in your life?* [focused open-ended inquiry]
> ***How*** *would you describe Buddy's job?* [focused open-ended inquiry]
> ***What*** *activities do you and Buddy like to do together?* [focused open-ended inquiry]

Past medical and surgical history: Elicit the full medical and surgical history of each new patient.

> ***From reviewing the records***, *it looks like Buddy was neutered at adoption, had a benign mass removed a couple of years ago, and has been diagnosed with skin allergies.* [internal summary] ***What*** *else should I know about him?* [open-ended inquiry]

Preventive medicine: Review the vaccination history; protocols for flea, tick, and heartworm prevention; and deworming schedule.

> ***What*** *do you recall about Buddy's vaccination history?* [focused open-ended inquiry]
> ***Tell me*** *about Buddy's vaccine plan.* [focused open-ended inquiry]
> ***What*** *oral or topical flea, tick, or heartworm preventive medications do you give Buddy?* [focused open-ended inquiry]

Nutrition: Conduct a full nutritional assessment of what and how the animal is fed. This includes the primary diet, treats, chews, table scraps, and indiscriminate eating habits.

> ***What*** *is Buddy's feeding routine?* [focused open-ended inquiry]
> ***Describe*** *for me everything Buddy eats in a day, starting from the beginning of the day to the end.* [focused open-ended inquiry]
> ***What*** *other things does Buddy eat?* [focused open-ended inquiry]

Medication and supplement history: Knowledge of a patient's medication and supplement history is crucial to avoid drug interactions, be aware of potential side effects, predict possible changes in laboratory tests, and to check for adherence. It is important to consider all medications: prescription and over-the-counter drugs, as well as natural and homeopathic remedies.

> *In addition to his food and treats,* ***what*** *else do you give Buddy?* [focused open-ended inquiry]
> ***What*** *medications is Buddy receiving now?* [focused open-ended inquiry]

> *What supplements do you give Buddy?* [focused open-ended inquiry]
> *What over-the-counter medications do you give Buddy?* [focused open-ended inquiry]

Pet's temperament and behavior: Ascertain the animal's personality, temperament, character, demeanor, and associated behaviors.

> *What is Buddy like at home with you?* [focused open-ended inquiry]
> *How would you describe Buddy's personality?* [focused open-ended inquiry]
> *What, if any, of Buddy's behaviors would you like to change?* [focused open-ended inquiry]

Client Data or Perspective

Understanding our clients' perspective and situation helps us relate to them and create a pragmatic long-term plan for the patient. Aspects of the client's perspective to explore include the client's ideas and beliefs, thoughts and feelings, knowledge and experiences, information preferences, occupation, and lifestyle. With increased societal recognition of the human–animal bond, it is helpful to explore the pet's acquisition story, and assess the client's level of attachment, caregiving roles and responsibilities in the household, and the impact of an animal's illness for each caregiver specifically.

Although it may not be possible to touch on all these issues with every client, it is important to gain insight into where the client is coming from. Eliciting information about the client's and others' viewpoints on the animal's illness fosters client participation and satisfaction and promotes shared decision-making. Doing so aids in identifying barriers to care and formulating a plan that fits best for the client, their pet, and their situation, potentiating buy-in and investment. Often, client- and/or environment-related factors are barriers to client acceptance of a recommendation.

Undoubtedly there will be times when we do not see eye to eye with our clients. In these moments, we show our support by acknowledging the client's point of view without necessarily agreeing with it. This nonjudgmental stance allows us to agree to disagree while respecting client autonomy. Acknowledgment lets the client know we hear them and recognize their views. These necessary steps create common ground through shared understanding.

> *It sounds like it is important to you that we address Buddy's discomfort.* [reflective listening – paraphrasing]
> *I'm concerned that the supplement you're providing may be hard on Buddy's kidneys and liver. Would you be open to discussing that further?* [closed-ended inquiry]
> *Would you consider discussing a change to Buddy's diet to one with joint support?* [closed-ended inquiry]

Acquisition of the pet: Request the pet's origin story, as it offers an opportunity to demonstrate interest in the client and their pet while gaining rich background as to how the client acquired the pet, informing possible genetic predispositions, potential exposure to previous risk factors, adverse events, or anticipated behavioral concerns.

> *How did Buddy come into your life?* [focused open-ended inquiry]

Client's level of attachment to the pet: There is evidence that the stronger the human–animal bond, the more likely clients are to follow a veterinarian's recommendation and seek preventive care for their animal(s) (Lue et al. 2008). The decision to follow a veterinarian's recommendation was associated with the client's understanding of the value of the veterinarian's recommendation and the client's attachment to their pet.

> ***How*** *would you describe your relationship with Buddy?* [focused open-ended inquiry]

Ideas and beliefs: Clients formulate ideas about what is going on with their animal. Validation of their beliefs and understanding, without necessarily agreeing with their ideas, is important in establishing the veterinarian-client-patient relationship.

> ***What*** *do you think is going on?* [focused open-ended inquiry]
> ***What*** *beliefs do you have about caring for Buddy that you'd like to share with me?* [focused open-ended inquiry]

Thoughts and feelings: Clients experience emotions, thoughts, and feelings as they cope with their animal's illness. They may be in shock or feel guilt, sadness, helplessness, grief, or anger. They may blame others or show signs of denial or acceptance, or they may be strong, silent, and stoic.

> ***What*** *are your thoughts?* [open-ended inquiry]
> ***How*** *are you doing?* [open-ended inquiry]
> ***How*** *do you think Buddy is doing?* [open-ended inquiry]
> ***How*** *do you feel about this?* [open-ended inquiry]

Knowledge and experiences: To gauge the entry point into the conversation, assess the client's starting knowledge and experiences using open-ended inquiry. Each client brings their own knowledge, background, and ideas to the table. Find out what the client already knows before delivering information to meet the client where they are.

> *You have cared for many dogs in your life.* [reflective listening – interpretation] ***What*** *experiences have you had with lameness?* [focused open-ended inquiry]
> ***You mentioned*** *earlier that you have a friend with a dog who'd torn a cruciate ligament.* [reflective listening – paraphrasing] ***Tell me*** *what they shared with you.* [focused open-ended inquiry]
> ***What*** *have you read or heard about torn cruciate ligaments* [focused open-ended inquiry]

Information preferences: Some clients are perfectly content with the big picture, while others prefer a highly detailed or even technical, clinical, or medical discussion. For some clients, receiving information is empowering; but for others, it is incapacitating because avoidance, denial, or minimizing may be their vital coping mechanisms (Stoewen et al. 2019). Be mindful of applying a one-size-fits-all approach to giving information or making assumptions that clients prefer the same amount of information as you do. Seeking the client's information preferences enables us to customize our explanation to a client's individual needs.

> *So I know how to best present the information for you,* ***would you prefer*** *the big picture or a highly detailed discussion?* [closed-ended inquiry]
> ***How*** *do you learn best?* [focused open-ended inquiry]
> ***Would it be*** *helpful if I drew a picture for you?* [closed-ended inquiry]

*For some clients, information can be empowering, and for others, it's overwhelming. **How** do you see yourself on that continuum?* [focused open-ended inquiry]

Occupation: The client's profession may frame, inform, or bias all the previous items, so it is helpful to know the client's background.

*As it may help me provide appropriate client education, **would you mind sharing** with me what you do for a living?* [closed-ended inquiry]
*Given your job, **what** is your lifestyle like?* [focused open-ended inquiry]

Client lifestyle (schedule, routine, and financial resources): The client's day-to-day lifestyle is likely tightly linked to their pet's care, activities, and routine. Explore how the client spends their time, what they like to do with their pet, or if they have any financial limitations or concerns.

***Walk me through** a typical day for you and Buddy.* [focused open-ended inquiry]
***Describe** your and Buddy's daily routine.* [focused open-ended inquiry]
***Tell me** your concerns about working these twice-daily treatments into your schedule.* [focused open-ended inquiry]
***What** were you anticipating financially for today's visit?* [focused open-ended inquiry]
***How** will these recommendations fit into your budget?* [focused open-ended inquiry]
***What** are your questions about the costs of today's visit?* [focused open-ended inquiry]

Pet caregivers' roles and responsibilities: Identify who is responsible for caring for the pet, their roles and responsibilities, and associated tasks, and assess the client's support system.

***Who** is responsible for taking care of Buddy at home?* [focused open-ended inquiry]
***What** responsibilities do they take on?* [focused open-ended inquiry]
***Tell me** about who takes care of Buddy when you are unable to do so.* [focused open-ended inquiry]

Impact of the pet's health on the animal's and clients' lives: The patient's health or illness often impacts the client's and the animal's function, day-to-day routine, and activities. Caregiver burden is associated with decreased psychosocial function for the client and increased reliance on veterinary services (Spitznagel et al. 2019). Clients experiencing caregiver burden face challenges in providing care for their animal due to the increased demands on their lifestyle and changes in their routine.

***How** has Buddy's lameness impacted your lives together?* [focused open-ended inquiry]
***What** has been most difficult for you and Buddy <ask about one at a time>?* [focused open-ended inquiry]
***How** is Buddy's lameness impacting you and others in your household <ask about one at a time>?* [focused open-ended inquiry]

Environment Data
Paint a picture of the animal's social interactions with people and other animals, the animal's daily routine, the household's lifestyle and schedule, and recent changes and life events to gain a greater understanding of the setting in which the client and animal live. Also evaluate the patient's level of risk and exposure by obtaining the animal's travel history (i.e. in and outside

the state/province or country) and local trips (i.e. hiking trails, walking in local parks, or playing in dog parks). It bears repeating that client or environmental factors are often barriers to accepting veterinarian recommendations.

Social interactions (human–human, human–animal, and animal–animal): A complete behavioral assessment includes painting a picture of how the animal interacts with other animals and people within and outside the household. Such information also determines the level of risk and exposure to environmental and infectious agents.

> **What** *other animals live in your household?* [focused open-ended inquiry]
> **Tell me** *about how everyone gets along.* [focused open-ended inquiry]
> **Who** *does Buddy socialize with outside of your home?* [focused open-ended inquiry]
> **Take me on a verbal tour** *of where you and Buddy go to play or exercise <ask about one at a time>.* [focused open-ended inquiry]
> **Who** *shares your home with you and Buddy?* [focused open-ended inquiry]
> **How** *do they interact with Buddy?* [focused open-ended inquiry]

Pet's activities of daily living (routine, feeding, exercise, sleeping habits, environmental enrichment, housing, and setting): A thorough description of the activities of daily living complements information gathered about the animal's role and function and the client's lifestyle. How well the animal is doing with these tasks and behaviors is critical to evaluating overall health, well-being, and quality of life.

> **Walk** *me through how Buddy spends a typical day.* [focused open-ended inquiry]
> **How** *has Buddy's lameness changed his exercise routine?* [focused open-ended inquiry]
> **Where** *does Buddy spend most of his time?* [focused open-ended inquiry]
> **How** *has Buddy been sleeping since the lameness started?* [focused open-ended inquiry]

Household lifestyle (schedule, routine, and travel): Understanding the interactions, activities, and daily routine of other household members is important because other people or animals play a role in the animal's health, wellness, and welfare.

> **Describe** *your home setting for me.* [focused open-ended inquiry]
> **Tell me** *about the places Buddy has traveled to in the past year.* [focused open-ended inquiry]
> **What** *does your household schedule look like?* [focused open-ended inquiry]
> **How** *does Buddy take part in household activities?* [focused open-ended inquiry]

Recent life events (marriage/divorce, new additions, construction/renovations, recent move, and job stability): Change is the crux of life, so take time during each visit to ask about any recent changes to the household. Such events are often stressful on the animal and may contribute to the illness.

> **What** *is new in your and Buddy's lives?* [focused open-ended inquiry]
> **What** *changes have occurred in your household or lifestyle since we last met <ask about one at a time>?* [focused open-ended inquiry]
> **How** *has that impacted you and Buddy <ask about one at a time>?* [focused open-ended inquiry]

Commonly Asked Questions Related to Information-Gathering

Why Make the Time to Gather a Complete History?

There are several thoughts to take into consideration regarding the time spent gathering data. The first is checking our perceptions of time, which are often inaccurate. In human medicine, most patients took less than 60 seconds to complete their opening statements, and none took longer than 150 seconds (Beckman and Frankel 1984). Similarly, in veterinary practice, it may feel like forever when the client is speaking; however, letting the client hold the floor yields higher-quality information (Research Spotlight 4.5).

Research Spotlight 4.5

How Long Do Clients Speak, and What Is Gained?

In the companion animal study examining veterinarians' solicitation of client concerns at the start of an appointment, clients spoke on average for 13 seconds following an open-ended solicitation and 5 seconds following a closed-ended solicitation. Yet in those additional 8 seconds, clients participating in the study shared significantly more concerns with their veterinarian following an open-ended solicitation (compared to the closed-ended approach) (Dysart et al. 2011).

Similarly, the study investigating the effect of different diet-history questions on gathering nutrition-related information from pet owners found that, following an open-ended inquiry, clients spoke on average for 44 seconds compared to 15 seconds after a closed-ended inquiry. For the additional 29 seconds, clients shared a significantly greater number of dietary items in response to the open-ended inquiry (average of 3.5 items) compared to the closed-ended inquiry (average of 1.3 items) (Coe et al. 2020). These results highlight that using open-ended inquiry does not take much longer, and it pays off by gathering significantly more information.

Taking time at the beginning of the clinical interview to gather the complete story about the patient, client, and environment pays off in a smooth diagnostic- and treatment-planning process. A full history minimizes the chances of a misdiagnosis and increases the chances of getting it right the first time, resulting in significant time savings for the veterinary team and cost savings for the client.

Using a conversational approach during information-gathering builds rapport and trust with the client. This results in critical buy-in to diagnostic or treatment recommendations. Gathering a complete history is a long-term investment strategy in building a relationship with the client and ensuring that the pet gets the care it needs.

What about Combining History Gathering and Performing the Physical Examination?

Some veterinary professionals combine history gathering with getting the temperature, pulse, respiration, weight, and body condition score or performing the entire physical exam. This dual-tasking approach may seem efficient, but it creates other challenges. Perceiving the veterinary professional as distracted, the client may not feel heard and, in frustration, may stop sharing information. Or the opposite may happen; clients repeat themselves because they felt they were not heard the first time. Both situations reduce efficiency.

By combining these two tasks, the veterinary professional may not fully explore the history relating to the patient, the client, and their environment or may overlook a physical exam finding. In addition, we are missing the opportunity to educate the client and communicate the value of the physical examination (da Costa et al. 2022). In human medicine, the history and physical examination were found to make up as much as 88% of diagnoses (Crombie 1963, Sandler 1980). Given this finding, the history and physical examination each deserve our undivided attention.

Can't I Focus on the History of the Animal Patient?

A complete history paves the path for client adherence to diagnostic and treatment plans. Common barriers to client adherence often reside in the client or environment domains of a history. Knowing the factors that may hinder a successful diagnostic or treatment plan enables you to develop a care plan specifically tailored to that client and their pet. Such a customized plan best fits the needs, desires, and abilities of the client and patient (Research Spotlight 4.6).

Research Spotlight 4.6

Basis for Client Resistance

Researchers observing veterinarians' conversations with pet owners about their pet's diet found that veterinarians' attempts to initiate proposals for long-term dietary changes were often met with client resistance. When the investigators explored the participating clients' basis for resistance after the veterinarian's proposal, they found it was often the result of patient- (e.g., food preferences) or environment-related (e.g., multi-pet households) information shared by clients (MacMartin, Wheat, and Coe, 2023). These findings highlight the importance of obtaining a complete history, including patient, client, and environment data prior to making a medical recommendation.

Where in the Interview Do I Gather the History?

Since the history guides the physical examination and lays the foundation for the diagnostic and treatment planning process, it is critical to grasp the full picture before moving forward. Investing up front in creating a precise history pays off in a more efficient diagnostic- and treatment-planning process. The end goal is to gather a complete and thorough history before moving on to the physical examination and the diagnostic and treatment plan.

Veterinary professionals commonly toggle back and forth between information-gathering and diagnostic and treatment planning. The potential consequences are sacrificing the structure of the interview, losing our train of thought, and missing key data or client concerns. Stay the course, remain disciplined, and note topics to come back to later.

Even with the best-laid plans, new information may arise later in the clinical interview. To maximize efficiency, check at multiple points during information-gathering to ensure that you fully elicited the client's goals, observations, and concerns, and then summarize for completeness.

Who on the Veterinary Team Gathers the History?

Today, information-gathering is often a team approach. It usually starts on the phone or at the reception desk when the client service coordinator or representative identifies the client's reason(s) for the appointment. Next, the veterinary technician gathers the initial history from the client. Then the veterinarian seeks additional information, filling in gaps and clarifying key details.

Who on the veterinary team gathers the history depends on the coordination of care between team members at each step. It involves the accurate transfer of information, meticulous record-keeping, and regular team-member briefings. To establish a reliable process, all veterinary team members require training on the important content pieces – patient, client, and environment – and the five communication skills for effective information-gathering. The goal is to share the knowledge, processes, and skills with the whole team to achieve efficient and accurate information-gathering.

To demonstrate continuity of team communication, the veterinarian summarizes for the client what they learned from the veterinary technician and other team members. Then the veterinarian uses an open-ended check to ensure what they heard was accurate (e.g. *What would you like to add?*) and asks for any key missing details (e.g. *What else do you think I should know about Buddy?*). With that foundation in place, the veterinarian poses clarifying questions to obtain a complete picture of the patient's current and previous history.

Why Didn't They Share That with Me?

A common frustration for members of the veterinary team after gathering the initial history is feeling that clients wait and reveal information only to the veterinarian. The team member may wonder, **Why is the client holding out on me?** However, the team member succeeded in their responsibilities; their initiation of information-gathering primes the pump for the client to remember key details. The veterinarian's inquiries offer a chance for clients to clarify or elaborate on their earlier responses.

During information-gathering, clients assess our willingness to listen, degree of interest, and level of care and compassion. Pay close attention to client verbal clues and nonverbal behaviors to pick up on concerns as they arise. When clients are invited to tell their full story and feel heard, a trusting relationship develops. Clients usually do not deliberately withhold information; they may be waiting for the "right time" or until they feel comfortable or safe enough to share the information with us.

Routine Client Scenario

Set the Scene: In response to Dr. Patel's question *Walk me through what's been going on with Buddy* [open-ended inquiry], Ms. Srinivasan shares, *Buddy's been lame since he slipped on the ice, and it seems to be worsening.*

> **Tell me** *more about Buddy's lameness.* [focused open-ended inquiry]
> **What** *did you notice when it first started?* [focused open-ended inquiry]
> **How** *has the lameness changed?* [focused open-ended inquiry]
> **How** *is Buddy's lameness* **impacting you**? [focused open-ended inquiry – client's perspective – effect of illness]
> **What** *do* **you think** *is going on?* [focused open-ended inquiry – client's perspective – thoughts]
> **How** *were* **you hoping** *we could address this today?* [focused open-ended inquiry – client's perspective – thoughts]
> **What I'm hearing is** *that it started when he slipped on the ice. He seemed to get better, and then after playing with another dog at the park, he got worse again. It started with limping, and now he is not using the leg at all.* [internal summary] **What** *would you like to add?* [open-ended inquiry]

Challenging Client Scenario

Set the Scene: In response to Dr. Patel's question *What do you think is going on?*, Ms. Srinivasan shares that based on her internet research, she believes Buddy tore his right cruciate ligament. She insists, without further workup, on referral to an orthopedic specialist for a TPLO (tibial plateau leveling osteotomy) surgery.

> *You're right; a* **torn cruciate ligament** *is one of the potential causes of Buddy's lameness.* [reflective listening – echoing]
> **What** *did you* **learn from your research** *about torn cruciate ligaments?* [focused open-ended inquiry – client's perspective – knowledge]

It sounds like you learned a lot, and your main concern is preventing arthritis in his knee with timely surgical correction. [reflective listening – paraphrase]

Would you be open to me conducting a complete physical and orthopedic examination on Buddy, so I can get a better sense of what's going on? [closed-ended inquiry]

Talk Through Technology – Use of Computers or Tablets in the Examination Room

The introduction of technology in the examination room (e.g. computer terminals, laptops, tablets, video screens, and smartphones) changes the dynamic of the veterinary professional–client interaction. As much as we need to be aware that these devices act as communication barriers, they also establish even greater partnerships. Here are some things to consider when integrating technology in the examination room to assist with information-gathering:

1. **Consider the placement of the computer screen or monitor**. When appropriate, position the screen so that both parties are privy to the information and view it together.

   Let's sit together here and look up Buddy's weight from previous visits.

   We can look up the date in Buddy's record together so we know for sure when we last evaluated his bloodwork.

2. **Take Notes**. Ask permission to take notes or make the client aware you are taking a brief break in the conversation to jot or type key details. This gives the client time to pause and reflect as well. Share notes with the client in the form of an internal summary to check their accuracy and engage the client in the note-taking process.

   So, I've written the lameness started in December. Initially, it was intermittent. Then, in February, it worsened and became a daily event, and you came in today because you're concerned that Buddy is no longer using his right leg. [internal summary] *What would you like to clarify?* [focused open-ended inquiry]

3. **Use a third-party recorder, dictation software, artificial intelligence, or note-taking tool**. Use technology or invite support staff to record notes during the visit so that the veterinary technician or veterinarian give the client their undivided attention without the distraction of capturing notes.

   Let me introduce you to Meera, who is going to take notes on our discussion in Buddy's medical record. [make introduction to the client and clarify your role]

   This new dictation program captures my notes. If it's all right with you, I'd like to summarize back what you've shared with me? [closed-ended inquiry] *Please listen and let me know if you have any corrections or clarifications.*

   I can save the notes I'm taking on my tablet directly into Buddy's medical record.

4. **Invite a third party into the conversation**. Invite the client to bring a member of their support team to join the conversation in person or using speakerphone or video call, to add additional information or perspective; this eliminates the need to repeat history-gathering with another family member.

   Would you like to call your partner so they can offer their observations? [closed-ended inquiry]

   Who else might be able to contribute key details on Buddy's lameness? [focused open-ended inquiry]

   How do you feel about inviting them to join us via the phone? [focused open-ended inquiry – client's perspective – feelings]

Gather Situation, Colleague, and Environment Information

As with client interactions, be intentional about how you gather information from colleagues. It is easy to leap to problem-solving and solution-generating before fully understanding the scope of the circumstances or issues. This means taking a step back to be curious, learn more, and explore the situation before coming to conclusions.

As veterinary medicine moves from a traditional paternalistic leadership approach, where the practice owner or hospital manager sets the agenda and leads it forward, to a partnership approach, the entire team is engaged in identifying priorities and involved in developing options. Our colleagues bring specialized skill sets, backgrounds, and experiences that enrich the exploration of potential paths. So, invite their expertise into the conversation to come up with various resolutions to challenging dilemmas – and give a sigh of relief that not everything is on the shoulders of practice leadership (Sidebar 4.9).

Sidebar 4.9   Team Outcomes of Effective Information-Gathering

Improve efficiency
Enhance satisfaction
Foster retention
Promote buy-in
Potentiate problem-solving
Generate creative solutions

Attend to the Process of Information-Gathering with Colleagues

It will not surprise you that the **how** of gathering colleague information uses the same five key communication skills outlined above. Use the inquiry funnel to start with broad, open-ended inquiries, move to focused open-ended inquiries, and finalize the details with closed-ended inquiries. Give plenty of space for colleagues to speak, and be mindful of interruptions. Signal that you are listening with minimal encouragers and reflective listening. Regularly, summarize what you heard to check for accuracy and pull the key details together.

Attend to the Content of Information-Gathering with Colleagues

The **what** of gathering information from colleagues includes exploring the situation, colleague's viewpoint, and environmental factors (Sidebar 4.10). The veterinary professional picks and chooses questions based on what they already know about the circumstances at hand, from interacting and working with colleagues, and what they need to know more about. The nature of the problem will guide which questions are most appropriate. The goal is to fully understand what is going on, what can be done about it, and what support, resources, and mentorship are required.

Note that we are not entitled to – nor are our colleagues obliged to – share personal or medical information. However, if they feel safe doing so, it puts us in a stronger position to advocate for, mentor, and offer confidential help and resources. Creating a professional and trusting relationship with colleagues provides a supportive backdrop, especially for sensitive conversations. So does modeling vulnerability, authenticity, and openness to break down barriers and stigmas.

Sidebar 4.10   The "What" of Colleague Information-Gathering

1. **Situation data**
   Sequence and progression of events
   Analysis of interactions
   Accountability
   Contributing factors
   Solutions tried

2. **Colleague data**
   a. **Colleague's perspective**
      Ideas and beliefs
      Thoughts and feelings
      Knowledge and experiences
      Information preferences
      Impact on work and home life

   b. **Professional background**
      Roles and responsibilities
      Educational and professional background
      Specialized training and certifications
      Communication, leadership, and professional skills
      Sources of motivation
      Performance evaluation
      Professional development plan
      Career goals

   c. **Personal wellness**
      Physical
      Spiritual
      Intellectual
      Environmental
      Financial
      Social
      Emotional
      Vocational

3. **Environment data**
   Lifestyle (household, schedule, routine, travel, and financial resources)
   Recent life events (marriage/divorce, new additions, construction/renovations, recent move)

Situation Data

First, in approaching any circumstance, paint a complete picture of the situation: what happened, how it occurred, who was involved, what contributed, what was attempted to resolve it, what the colleague's role was, and what assistance they need. For solutions to be successful, start with the full story; appreciating the complexity of the situation may require conversations with multiple individuals. Be mindful of our natural tendency to move quickly to find it and fix it, as a fast solution may not be a smart, long-term, or sustainable one.

Examples

> **Share** *with me from the beginning what happened.* [open-ended inquiry]
> **What** *happened next?* [focused open-ended inquiry]
> **Who** *was involved?* [focused open-ended inquiry]
> **What** *role did you play?* [focused open-ended inquiry]
> **What** *have you tried to resolve it so far?* [focused open-ended inquiry]
> **What** *kind of support would you like from me?* [focused open-ended inquiry]
> **What** *resources might you need from the practice?* [focused open-ended inquiry]

Colleague Data

Gathering colleague information includes exploring their perspective, professional background, and personal wellness.

Colleague's Perspective

Although it may not be possible to touch on all these issues with every colleague, it is important to gain insight into where the individual is coming from. Our colleagues bring their unique outlooks to the table – their ideas and beliefs, thoughts and feelings, knowledge and experiences, information preferences, and understanding of the impact on their work and home life. They possess a distinct viewpoint and therefore are poised to offer alternative approaches. Seeing a scenario from multiple vantage points allows for more creative strategies and innovative outcomes.

Examples

> **What** *factors do you think contributed to the situation?* [focused open-ended inquiry]
> **How** *are you feeling about it?* [focused open-ended inquiry]
> **What** *would you like to see happen?* [focused open-ended inquiry]
> **How** *do you think we should handle it?* [focused open-ended inquiry]
> **What** *experiences do you have in this realm?* [focused open-ended inquiry]
> **How** *is this situation impacting you?* [focused open-ended inquiry]
> **How** *is this affecting your work / home life <ask one at a time>?* [focused open-ended inquiry]

Professional Background

To prepare for a conversation with a colleague, review the colleague's background and employment history. Note what information is well-documented and what areas need further exploration.

Examples

> **What** *expertise can you bring to this situation?* [focused open-ended inquiry]
> **What** *training might you need to tackle this?* [focused open-ended inquiry]
> **How** *might we incorporate this into your professional development plan?* [focused open-ended inquiry]
> **What** *motivates you to take this on?* [focused open-ended inquiry]
> **How** *will this impact your career trajectory?* [focused open-ended inquiry]

Personal wellness

Eight dimensions of personal wellness have been identified: physical, spiritual, intellectual, environmental, financial, social, emotional, and vocational (Hettler 1976, Stoewen 2017). Consider and explore these eight aspects of optimal health and well-being with colleagues. Take time to discover what might be going on internally for them – ask about self-care, social support, learning disabilities, mental health issues, eating or sleep disorders, or substance abuse. If concerned about a colleague's well-being, be prepared to provide or refer to mental health community resources, such as employee assistance programs, regional or national veterinary association resources, and crisis or suicide hotlines.

Examples

> **How** *do you feel about your self-care?* [focused open-ended inquiry]
> **What** *do you do to take care of yourself?* [focused open-ended inquiry]
> **What** *do you like to do physically?* [focused open-ended inquiry]
> **Describe** *how spirituality fits into your life?* [focused open-ended inquiry]
> **How** *do you like to challenge your mind?* [focused open-ended inquiry]
> **Share with me** *how your home/work environment <ask one at a time> support your well-being?* [focused open-ended inquiry]
> **What** *kind of financial pressures are you facing?* [focused open-ended inquiry]
> **Tell me about** *your social outlets?* [focused open-ended inquiry]
> **Who** *do you turn to for emotional support?* [focused open-ended inquiry]
> **How** *does this position fit into your values, goals, and lifestyle <ask one at a time>? [focused open-ended inquiry]*
> **How** *do you manage your stress?* [focused open-ended inquiry]
> **What** *help are you seeking for your depression or anxiety?* [focused open-ended inquiry]

Environment Data

In exploring colleague environmental factors, ascertain what is happening at work and at home to determine what may play a role in a colleague's reaction or perspective. Although we strive to leave home at home, the reality is that these demands creep into the workplace. And likewise, it is equally challenging not to bring our work home with us.

Examples

> **What** *is happening at home that may be impacting your work?* [focused open-ended inquiry]
> **How** *is your work impacting your home life?* [focused open-ended inquiry]
> **What** *does your daily routine look like?* [focused open-ended inquiry]
> **What's** *changed for you at home?* [focused open-ended inquiry]

Veterinary professionals who read this may think, **this is none of my business**. But if it impacts our business, it is our business. And with growing concerns for professional wellness, it is our professional responsibility to care for our colleagues; provide an open, safe, and nonjudgmental space to conduct these conversations; and identify and provide support and resources – not just for the success of our practice but also for the entire veterinary profession.

Routine Team Scenario

Set the scene: Dalia, the practice manager, recently released the new team schedule, which was received with complaints and dissatisfaction. So, she calls a team meeting to better understand the team's concerns.

> **How** *are you all doing?* [open-ended inquiry]
> **What is working for all of you** *with the current scheduling process?* [focused open-ended inquiry – colleague's perspective – experiences]

> **It sounds like** we agree that it's a fair process, and everyone is getting the hours they need. [internal summary]
>
> I'm curious – **what** is most disagreeable to you about this schedule? [focused open-ended inquiry – colleague's perspective – thoughts]
>
> **The biggest challenge seems** to be planning for last-minute absences due to illnesses or family emergencies. [reflective listening – paraphrasing]
>
> **What ideas** do you have for developing a backup system for clinic coverage? [focused open-ended inquiry – colleague's perspective – ideas]
>
> How do **you think** we can implement that? [focused open-ended inquiry – colleague's perspective – thoughts]

Challenging Team Scenario

Set the scene: The phone is ringing off the hook. Dalia, the practice manager, is walking through the waiting room to greet a client and overhears Meera, one of the client service coordinators, asking Stacey, a veterinary technician, if she might pick up one of the calls. Stacey replies, *"That's not my job."*

> Stacey, **I'm wondering if** we can talk for a few minutes. [closed-ended inquiry]
>
> I overheard an interaction between you and Meera this morning when the phones were ringing off the hook. **I heard you say** that it was **not your job** to answer the phones. [reflective listening – echoing]
>
> **Would you share with me** what was going on for you? [open-ended inquiry – colleague's perspective – experiences]
>
> **What** do you see as your responsibilities? [focused open-ended inquiry – colleague's perspective – beliefs]
>
> **How** can we work together to overcome this as a team? [focused open-ended inquiry – colleague's perspective – ideas]
>
> **How** do you think we can make that happen? [focused open-ended inquiry – colleague's perspective – thoughts]

Put the Information-Gathering Skills into Practice

Do-It-Yourself Exercises

Exercise 4.1   Skill Spot – Question Type

Review the following example questions and indicate whether each is an open- or closed-ended inquiry. The answer key is at the end of the chapter.

1. *Is Buddy's lameness in the right front leg?*

2. *How has Buddy's lameness progressed over time?*

3. *How might we cover emergencies?*

4. *Does Buddy want to go for walks right now?*

5. *What improves Buddy's lameness?*

6. *Do we need to designate a colleague for emergency backup?*

Exercise 4.2 Skill Practice – Reflect Back

Read the following client or colleague statements and write a reflective listening statement in response. Suggested answers are provided at the end of the chapter.

1. *I am really concerned that Buddy tore his cruciate ligament. I read about it on the internet, and he is showing all the signs.*

2. *It all started when Buddy slipped on the ice. He took quite a fall, and his back legs just slipped right out from beneath him.*

3. *We are so short-staffed that everyone is scheduled full out, so there is no one available for backup if someone gets sick or in an emergency.*

Exercise 4.3 Self-Assessment

Depending on your practice role, you might want to self-reflect on a client or colleague conversation. Begin working on the five communication skills introduced in this chapter followed by self-assessment. Conduct a quick litmus test after a recent appointment or meeting using the following guiding questions.

1. What was my overall approach: conversational or interrogative?

2. How did I invite my client or colleague to share their ideas, thoughts, feelings, experiences, concerns, or expectations?

3. Being honest with myself, what interruptions did I note during the conversation? What was the consequence?

4. How did I pull together (summarize) the key details for myself and my client or colleague?

Exercise 4.4 Next Steps for Success

1. Based on what you learned from the previous self-assessment exercise, identify growth opportunities and prioritize the order in which you would like to work on the five communication skills introduced in this chapter.

2. Focus on one skill for a solid week. Note the results; then, the following week, work on another skill to broaden your information-gathering repertoire.

3. Identify a coaching partner in the practice: inform them of your communication goal, invite them to observe your interactions, and request specific, descriptive, and balanced feedback.

4. Be gentle and kind to yourself; trying new communication skills is awkward at first and takes effort until they become automatic.

5. Repeat the cycle of focusing on one communication skill, practice, and request feedback from a colleague or self-assess until you achieve competence with all five communication skills introduced in this chapter.

Engage-the-Entire-Team Exercises

Exercise 4.5   Twenty Questions (Coe 2017)

1. Choose a simple picture from the internet or a book with several inanimate objects in the background, and keep it concealed from the team.

2. Identify an activity facilitator who does the following:
   a. Keeps track of time
   b. Observes and identifies question types
   c. Counts the number of questions asked

3. Identify two volunteers:
   a. **Visionary:** Is given the picture and does not show it to anyone else; responds to questions posed by the team
   b. **Artist:** Draws the picture on a flipchart, whiteboard, or chalkboard based on what is learned from the team's questions

4. Round one – 20 closed-ended inquiries:
   a. Invite the team to ask the Visionary 20 yes/no questions about the picture.
   b. The Visionary responds with only yes/no answers.
   c. The Artist attempts to draw the picture based on the questions asked by the team and the Visionary's yes or no responses.
   d. Debrief the activity, but do not disclose the original picture yet:
      i. How long did it take?
      ii. What was drawn by the Artist?

5. Round two – open-ended inquiry:
   a. Invite the team to ask the Visionary one broad, inviting, open-ended inquiry about the picture.
   b. Pay attention, and ask the team to reframe the proposed inquiry if it is closed-ended or a focused open-ended inquiry.
   c. Once a broad, inviting, open-ended inquiry is proposed (e.g. *Tell me . . ., Describe . . .*), the Visionary responds with an appropriate multi-sentence description.
   d. Finish with the Visionary disclosing the original picture to the team.

6. Debrief the exercise:
   a. How much time did each approach take?
   b. What was the impact of asking 20 closed inquiries versus one open-ended inquiry?

c. Which approach gathered more information about the original picture?

d. How does this translate to information-gathering with clients or hearing a colleague's concerns?

7. Conclude by reviewing the Inquiry Funnel (Figure 4.1) with the team.

Exercise 4.6 Back-Pocket, Open-Ended Inquiries to Ask Clients

1. As a team, brainstorm 10 open-ended inquiries (e.g. about the patient, client's perspective, and environment) that could be asked during every appointment, no matter the client, patient, or presentation.

2. Pay close attention, listen for closed-ended examples (i.e. yes/no), and work as a team to rephrase them into open-ended inquiries (e.g. *Tell me, Describe, Elaborate, Explain, What,* or *How*).

3. Your team now owns a list of carefully crafted back-pocket questions to work with. Post this list of questions in your electronic medical record, place them on your clipboard, or hang them on the back of the examination room door as a reminder to implement them during information-gathering.

4. Ask each team member to focus on one of these open-ended inquiries and practice the question or statement until it becomes second nature during information-gathering. Encourage them to practice to the point where they no longer think about asking open-ended inquiry – it just happens!

Exercise 4.7 Revisit the Practice's History Checklist

1. In light of the information-gathering lessons in this chapter, reexamine as a team or in small groups the practice's history checklist most likely posted in your electronic medical record.

2. Look at each item and identify how the question is posed (open versus closed-ended inquiry).

3. Rephrase closed-ended to open-ended inquiry and revise the practice history checklist. Most questions can be couched as an open-ended inquiry to obtain the information we are seeking.

Take It Away

1. Be curious and use **open-ended inquiry** to hear your client's or colleague's full story – to envision the situation as if you were there – and **closed-ended inquiry** to clarify finer details and fill in the final puzzle pieces.

2. Gather an understanding of your **client's or colleague's perspective:** acknowledge their ideas and beliefs, knowledge and experiences, thoughts and feelings, as well as preferences

while gathering the information needed to care for your patient or solve colleague or team challenges.

3. **Pause** (three or more seconds) to allow time for all parties to process and assimilate information, determine what information is missing, and reflect on how to respond.

4. Use **minimal encouragers** (*Oh, Wow, Yeah, Uh-huh*) to invite your client or colleague to continue to share their story, thoughts, or feelings.

5. **Reflect** back what you heard to check the accuracy of the data-collection process, so clients or colleagues feel valued and heard, or to encourage elaboration.

Answer Key

Exercise 4.1   Skill Spot – Question Type

1. *Is Buddy's lameness in the right front leg?* [closed-ended inquiry]

2. *How has Buddy's lameness progressed over time?* [focused open-ended inquiry]

3. *How might we cover emergencies?* [focused open-ended inquiry]

4. *Does Buddy want to go for walks right now?* [closed-ended inquiry]

5. *What improves Buddy's lameness?* [focused open-ended inquiry]

6. *Do we need to designate a colleague for emergency backup?* [closed-ended inquiry]

Exercise 4.2   Skill Practice – Reflect Back

1. *I am really concerned that Buddy tore his cruciate ligament. I read about it on the internet, and he is showing all the signs.*
   Reflective listening: ***You're concerned it may be serious: that Buddy tore his cruciate ligament***. [echoing]

2. *It all started when Buddy slipped on the ice. He took quite a fall, and his back legs just slipped right out from beneath him.*
   Reflective listening: ***Sounds like a bad fall, and Buddy may have injured himself then***. [paraphrasing]

3. *We are so short-staffed that everyone is scheduled full out, so there is no one available for backup if someone gets sick or in an emergency.*
   Reflective listening: ***You're concerned that we don't have staff available to cover for unexpected schedule changes***. [paraphrasing]

References

Beckman, H.B. and Frankel, R.M. (1984). The effect of physician behavior on the collection of patient data. *Ann. Intern. Med.* 101 (5): 692–696. https://doi.org/10.7326/0003-4819-101-5-692.

Coe, J.B. (2017). Lunch and learn guide: Open-ended inquiry. Coe Consulting.

Coe, J.B., O'Connor, R.E., MacMartin, C. et al. (2020). Effects of three diet history questions on the amount of information gained from a sample of pet owners in Ontario, Canada. *J. Am. Vet. Med. Assoc.* 256 (4): 469–478. https://doi.org/10.2460/javma.256.4.469.

da Costa, J.C., Coe, J.B., Blois, S.L., and Stone, E.A. (2022). Veterinarians' use of the talking physical exam as a communication tool. *J. Am. Vet. Med. Assoc.* 260 (12): 1–8. https://doi.org/10.2460/javma.22.01.0048.

Crombie, D.L. (1963). Diagnostic process. *J. Coll. Gen. Pract.* 6 (4): 579–589.

Dysart, L.M., Coe, J.B., and Adams, C.L. (2011). Analysis of solicitation of client concerns in companion animal practice. *J. Am. Vet. Med. Assoc.* 238 (12): 1609–1615. https://doi.org/10.2460/javma.238.12.1609.

Groopman, J. (2007). *How Doctors Think*. New York, NY: Houghton Mifflin Company.

Hettler, B. (1976). *Six Dimensions of Wellness Model*. National Wellness Institute. www.nationalwellness.org (accessed 27 November 2023).

Kurtz, S., Silverman, J., Benson, J., and Draper, J. (2003). Marrying content and process in clinical method teaching: Enhancing the Calgary-Cambridge Guides. *Acad. Med.* 78 (8): 802–809. https://doi.org/10.1097/00001888%2D200308000%2D00011.

MacMartin, C., Wheat, H.C., Coe, J.B., and Adams, C.L. (2015). Effect of question design on dietary information solicited during veterinarian-client interactions in companion animal practice in Ontario, Canada. *J. Am. Vet. Med. Assoc.* 246 (11): 1203–1214. https://doi.org/10.2460/javma.246.11.1203.

MacMartin, C., Wheat, H.C., and Coe, J.B. (2023). Conversation Analysis of Clients' Active Resistance to Veterinarians' Proposals for Long-Term Dietary Change in Companion Animal Practice in Ontario, Canada. *Animals* 13 (13): 1–39. https://doi.org/10.3390/ani13132150.

Sandler, G. (1980). The importance of the history in the medical clinic and the costs of unnecessary tests. *Am. Heart J.* 100 (6): 928–931. https://doi.org/10.1016/0002-8703(80)90076-9.

Shaw, J.R., Adams, C.L., Bonnett, B.N. et al. (2004). Use of the Roter interaction analysis system to analyze veterinarian-client-patient communication in companion animal practice. *J. Am. Vet. Med. Assoc.* 225 (2): 222–229. https://doi.org/10.2460/javma.2004.225.222.

Spitznagel, M.B., Cox, M.D., Jacobson, D.M. et al. (2019). Assessment of caregiver burden and associations with psychosocial function, veterinary service, use, and factors related to treatment plan adherence among owners of dogs and cats. *J. Am. Vet. Med. Assoc.* 254 (1): 124–132. https://doi.org/10.2460/javma.254.1.124.

Stoewen, D.L. (2017). Dimensions of wellness: Change your habits, change your life. *Can. Vet. J. V.* 58 (8): 861–862.

Stoewen, D.L., Coe, J.B., MacMartin, C. et al. (2019). Identification of illness uncertainty in veterinary oncology: implications for service. *Front. Vet. Sci.* 6: 147. https://doi.org/10.3389/fvets.2019.00147.

5

Attending to Relationships

Abstract

In day to day work with clients and colleagues, we walk a tightrope between creating connections and getting tasks done. The greatest barrier is finding and making time for relationship building. In this chapter, we tackle this balancing act, as spending too much time on either relationship-building or attending to tasks is detrimental to overall productivity, client service, patient care, professional satisfaction, and teamwork. We introduce communication tools that strive for a middle ground; that construct a friendly, caring, supportive clinical setting; and that build a goal-oriented, collaborative veterinary team. A highly functional team meets the appointment, treatment, and surgical schedules; supports each other; and provides high-quality patient care and compassionate client care. In this chapter, we explore four key communication skills that attend to relationships with clients and colleagues: nonverbal behaviors, empathy, partnership, and asking permission.

SELF-ASSESSMENT QUESTIONS

1. What is my natural tendency: to focus on building relationships or completing tasks?
2. How attuned am I to the feelings of others when reading and interpreting their nonverbal and verbal cues?
3. How do I intentionally approach communication to build relationships with clients or colleagues?
4. How does my relationship-building communication differ with clients versus colleagues?

Introduction

This book led with communication styles as the broader framework in which relationships are viewed. The communication style employed in an interaction drives how the communication skills are used. The expert style is more invested in getting tasks done, while the partner style values collaboration and consensus-building.

In day to day work with clients and colleagues, we walk a tightrope between creating connections and getting tasks done. This is a balancing act, as spending too much time on either relationship-building or attending to tasks is detrimental to overall productivity, client service, patient care,

Developing Communication Skills for Veterinary Practice, First Edition. Jane R. Shaw and Jason B. Coe.
© 2024 John Wiley & Sons, Inc. Published 2024 by John Wiley & Sons, Inc.

professional satisfaction, and teamwork. We introduce communication tools that strive for a middle ground to construct a friendly, caring, supportive clinical setting and build a goal-oriented, collaborative veterinary team. A highly functional team meets the appointment, treatment, and surgical schedules; supports each other; and provides high-quality patient care and compassionate client care.

The most common rebuttal is, **"I don't have time for this relationship stuff. It takes too much time."** Given our daily demands, it is easy to focus on tasks, and doing so erodes client and team relationships. The greatest barrier is finding and making the time for relationship-building in day to day practice. Therefore, take timeouts, even scheduled ones, to attend to relationships with self, clients, and colleagues. The motivation to do so is that relational communication skills build trust and rapport with clients, grow team morale, engender our own satisfaction and fulfillment, and foster a great place to work (Sidebar 5.1).

Sidebar 5.1   Clinical Outcomes of Attending to Relationships

Foster client satisfaction
Enhance data-gathering
Improve efficiency of interactions
Promote adherence
Reduce client complaints
Minimize malpractice claims

In this chapter, we explore four key communication skills that attend to relationships with clients or colleagues: nonverbal behaviors, empathy, partnership, and asking permission (Sidebar 5.2). We provide examples of these skills in two settings: in the examination room, working with Mr. Fitzgerald and Chloe; and in the treatment room, where Dr. Howell and Julie, the veterinary technician, work together to address the needs of a patient in an emergency.

Sidebar 5.2   Four Communication Skills for Attending to Relationships

Nonverbal behaviors
Empathy
Partnership
Asking permission

Set the Scene

Client Scenario: Mr. Fitzgerald presents to Dr. Howell with Chloe, a three-year-old female spayed domestic-short-hair cat that was recently rescued from the local shelter. Everyone, especially Julie, the veterinary technician, is pleased to see Mr. Fitzgerald, who is a "regular" at the clinic. Over the years, the practice cared for five of Mr. Fitzgerald's beloved and doted-on cats. Unfortunately, Chloe is urinating outside of the litterbox in her new home (Hunter and Shaw 2012).

Team Scenario: A patient in an emergency arrives at the hospital while Dr. Howell is presenting diagnostic options to Mr. Fitzgerald to rule out a medical problem for Chloe's inappropriate urination. Julie and Dr. Howell triage how to take care of the emergency patient and wrap up Mr. Fitzgerald's and Chloe's appointment.

Stepping into Dr. Howell's and Julie's shoes, self-reflect on:

1. How would I put Mr. Fitzgerald and Chloe at ease, given this stressful situation?
2. How would I team up with Dr. Howell to care for the needs of both patients?

Attend to Client Relationships

Key Communication Skills for Attending to Client Relationships

Nonverbal Behaviors

Definition
Physical expressions that accompany language use (Box 5.1). Pay attention to five sets of cues: kinesics (i.e. body movements and gestures), proxemics (i.e. spatial relationships), paralanguage (i.e. vocal qualities and cues), autonomic responses (i.e. uncontrolled reactions), and environmental cues (i.e. clinical environment, physical presentation (Research Spotlight 5.1), and emotional atmosphere). Demonstrations of nonverbal behaviors differ based on the clinical setting and appointment context (Research Spotlight 5.2).

Box 5.1 Five Types of Nonverbal Communication

1. **Kinesics**
   a. **Touch**: Handshake, pat on the arm, or a hug
   b. **Body movements:** Hand and arm gestures, nodding, fidgeting, foot and leg actions
   c. **Facial expressions**: Smile, frown, furrowed or raised eyebrows
   d. **Eye contact:** Gazing, staring, or avoiding
   e. **Posture:** Sitting, standing, slouching, or leaning
   f. **Body tension:** Arms relaxed/crossed, tight jawline, shoulders, or neck

2. **Proxemics**
   a. **Proximity:** Space and positioning between ourselves and the other person
   b. **Barriers:** Pet, examination table, carrier, computer, or furniture

3. **Paralanguage:** Pitch, rate, volume, rhythm, intonation, and emphasis

4. **Autonomic**: Tearing, blushing, blanching, sweating, breathing, pupil changes, and swallowing

5. **Environmental**
   a. **Physical presence:** Clothing, grooming, and cleanliness (Research Spotlight 5.1)
   b. **Environment:** Location, crowding, furniture placement, lighting, temperature, colors, odors, and cleanliness
   c. **Emotional atmosphere:** Anger, fear, pain, joy, passion, love, shame, or guilt

Adapted from Mehrabian (1972); Carson (2007); Hunter and Shaw (2012).

Research Spotlight 5.1

Veterinarian Attire Matters

In a study investigating the effects of veterinarian attire on pet owner ratings of trust, confidence, and comfort, participant scores were highest when the model veterinarian was pictured in surgical scrubs and lowest when they were wearing a casual shirt and blue jeans (Coe et al. 2020). Attire is a form of nonverbal communication that may also affect veterinary professional–client relationships, so being attentive to this communication and developing a practice-based dress code may be helpful.

Research Spotlight 5.2

Nonverbal Affect Differs in Preventive Care and Health Problem Appointments

In a study comparing veterinarian–client–patient communication in preventive care versus health-problem appointments, veterinarians sounded significantly more hurried in health-problem appointments than in preventive care appointments. Clients appeared to be significantly more anxious, nervous, and emotionally distressed or upset during problem appointments than in preventive care appointments (Shaw et al. 2008). These findings highlight the need for veterinary professionals to be aware and respond to their own and their client's nonverbal behaviors, especially during concerning and stressful health-problem appointments.

It is estimated that 80% of communication consists of implicit nonverbal signals and 20% is explicit verbal messages (Mehrabian 1971). Given their predominance, read nonverbal cues to bridge the gap between what is said and what is meant. Nonverbal behaviors make or break verbal expressions.

When nonverbal behaviors align with the content of the verbal message, the impact is enhanced, whereas when nonverbal and verbal cues are misaligned, the nonverbal message trumps the verbal statement. Because some nonverbal behaviors are unconscious, thoughts or feelings may "leak out" through our nonverbal channel and be seen by others as the truth. Nonverbal communication is powerful, associated with a number of outcomes of veterinary care (Research Spotlight 5.3), and influenced by communication training (Research Spotlight 5.4).

Research Spotlight 5.3

An Empathetic and Unhurried Affect Enhances Adherence

In a study investigating client adherence to dental and surgical recommendations, a more empathetic veterinarian and client tone and a less rushed veterinarian and client tone during visits were significantly associated with clients' adherence to the recommendation (Kanji et al. 2012). These results emphasize the importance of attending to veterinary professional and client nonverbal behavior during interactions, given their role in the outcomes of veterinary care.

Research Spotlight 5.4

Communication Training Fosters Positive Nonverbal Affect

In a study of communication education onsite in a veterinary practice, after training, veterinarian interest and attentiveness toward the client significantly increased, as did client interest and attentiveness, client friendliness and warmth, and client interactivity (Shaw et al. 2010).

In a similar study with another veterinary practice, both veterinarians and clients appeared significantly less hurried and veterinarians seemed significantly more empathetic toward clients after training (Shaw et al. 2012). Investing in training and providing opportunities for observation, feedback, and rehearsal enhances nonverbal affect during veterinary professional interactions.

Techniques

Two tasks are related to effective nonverbal communication:

1. Be aware of and respond to the nonverbal behaviors of others (Box 5.1). This requires:
   a. Be fully present to enhance attentive and perceptual abilities.
   b. Read the other person's nonverbal cues.
   c. Check out your interpretation of the nonverbal behaviors for accuracy.

   We rely solely on nonverbal behaviors to assess our animal patients. To determine how they are feeling and how to best approach our patients. We detect their posture, mentation, gait, responses, eyes, ears, head and tail carriage, and facial expressions. So, apply the same astute observational skills to perceive client's nonverbal signals.

   > **MR. FITZGERALD:** *I am concerned about Chloe's urinary accidents in the house. <He is visibly shaking, and before he breaks eye contact, his eyes are watering.>*
   > **DR. HOWELL:** *I see that you've grown quite attached to Chloe, and her inappropriate urination is upsetting for you.*

2. Enhance awareness of our nonverbal behaviors and how they are perceived by others (Box 5.1). As we are often "blind" to our nonverbal behaviors, these insights come from self-observation, video recording, and feedback from others.

   In the previous scenario, Mr. Fitzgerald may perceive Dr. Howell's response differently, depending on her nonverbal presentation (Hunter and Shaw 2012):
   a. If Dr. Howell speaks with a shaky and barely audible voice, with her eyes gazing downward, Mr. Fitzgerald may suspect a lack of confidence.
   b. If Dr. Howell stands upright, with an open posture, and looks Mr. Fitzgerald in the eye while using a confident tone of voice at an appropriate volume, he may feel supported and reassured.

Touch as a nonverbal expression deserves special mention and a word of caution. Although touch is a poignant way of connecting with others, it may not be appropriate or comfortable. Touch "safe zones" are the hand and forearm. If uncertain, ask permission, such as *Would it be all right if I offered you a hug?* If uncomfortable with touch, do not attempt it, as the client will perceive the discomfort. Close the distance without using touch by shifting closer, reaching out a hand, or touching the arm of the chair.

Empathy

Definition

Express an understanding and appreciation of a situation from another person's perspective. Set your point of view aside, and sense what this situation is like for them. Show empathy to connect with others; acknowledge, validate, and legitimize what the other person is going through (Box 5.2).

Box 5.2   Uses of Empathy

1. Acknowledge the other person

   *It sounds like your relationship with Chloe has gotten off to a **challenging** start.*

2. Legitimize or normalize their feelings

   *What may be making this more **stressful** is that you sense your options are limited.*

3. Appreciate the other person

   *Thank you for sharing that with me. It was **difficult** to share your greatest fear of losing her.*

4. Create a nonjudgmental setting

   *It seems like you may have been **worried** that I might judge you for considering rehoming Chloe as an option.*

Adapted from Hunter and Shaw (2012).

Technique

Empathy is expressed in three ways: nonverbal signals, verbal acknowledgment, or self-disclosure.

1. **Demonstrate nonverbal empathy:**
   a. Concerned facial expression; leaning in with attentive, soft eye contact
   b. Sitting in silence beside someone until they are ready to speak
   c. Reaching out with a hand, placing a hand on the arm of the chair, or offering a hug
   d. Shedding a tear in grief
   e. Clapping, jumping, or exclaiming joy in celebration
   f. Matching an urgent tone, short sentences, and quickened speech in an emergency
   g. Sighing, frowning, or furrowing the brow in frustration at a situation.

2. **Offer empathy as a verbal acknowledgment,** which involves two steps:

   Step 1: Perceive and identify the other's emotions (e.g. happiness, contentment, disappointment, frustration, guilt, sadness, anger, fright, anxiety, or hesitation) or experience (i.e. predicament, dilemma, or situation). In the previous scenario, if Mr. Fitzgerald is visibly shaking and his eyes are watering, he may be feeling upset, scared, anxious, overwhelmed, or sad.

   Step 2: Verbally express empathy by using an empathy stem, naming the emotion, and identifying the experience. (Sidebar 5.3). Be as specific, descriptive, and detailed as possible so the client feels seen and heard by you. To expand your emotional repertoire, consult the internet for lists of feeling words.

I sense your **attachment** already to Chloe, and you're **concerned** about what might happen if we cannot stop her urinary accidents in a timely manner. [empathy]

Sidebar 5.3 Empathy Stems

Finish these statements by naming the emotion you heard, saw, or understood and then stating the other person's predicament:

> *I appreciate that . . .*
> *I see that . . .*
> *I hear that . . .*
> *I sense that . . .*
> *It seems like . . .*
> *It sounds like . . .*
> *I understand . . .*
> *I can imagine . . .*

Consider honing in on empathy statements that target the client's specific predicament. Blanket empathy statements tend to be less effective; they are general and cover all situations, such as *I know you're going through a lot* or *That must be hard* or *That's frustrating*. Tailored empathy statements hit the target on the nose, such as *You're worried that Chloe's behavior may prevent her from being a member of your family*.

Expressing empathy by saying *I understand* deserves special consideration. The risk with using *I understand* is that clients may respond with *There is no way you understand what I am going through*, which is undoubtedly true. So, avoid stepping in the client's shoes (e.g. *I understand how much this is impacting you*), and be more explicit in stating exactly what was heard about the situation. For example, *I understand Chloe means a lot to you and you will do all you can to keep her in your family*.

3. **Empathize by revealing personal experiences.** Self-disclosure entails sharing a story that mirrors that of the other person to normalize the situation and relate and connect with them. A word of caution: the risk of self-disclosure is turning the spotlight on the veterinary professional. Maintain the focus on the client. To do so, keep sharing short, sweet, and to the point, and then direct the conversation back to the client.

   Our family came close to rehoming one of our cats due to inappropriate urination, and it was heartbreaking for us. [empathy] *We will work together to explore all of the options for you and Chloe.*

To enhance the impact of all forms of empathy, punctuate expressions with a long pause. This period of silence allows the empathy to sink in; provides the client time to reflect, process, and say more; and creates a shared emotional space. Additionally, a moment of contemplation and support diffuses client emotions and fosters their readiness to move forward with decision-making.

Research indicates that empathy is underutilized in veterinary appointments (McArthur and Fitzgerald 2013; Shaw et al. 2004) (Research Spotlight 5.5). To put this into perspective, researchers in human medicine report there are an average of 2.49 empathetic opportunities per physician–patient encounter (Bylund and Makoul 2002). Considering the celebratory, transformative, and emotional events in clients' lives, there are multiple windows of opportunity for verbal empathy in veterinary practice.

Research Spotlight 5.5

Lack of Verbal Expressions of Empathy

In a detailed analysis of veterinarian–client–patient communication in 150 preventive care and 150 health-related problem appointments in Canada, verbal empathy was expressed in 7% of appointments (Shaw et al. 2004). Opportunities remain for veterinary teams to use verbal empathy to support, connect with, and build trust with their clients and patients.

Given that clients perceive veterinarians to be kind, thoughtful, caring, and compassionate (Cron et al. 2000), it is clear veterinary professionals are empathetic. The concern is that we may preferentially express empathy nonverbally. Take time to also connect with clients by verbally empathizing directly with them. Empathy can be taught, and expressions of empathy increased after communication training (Research Spotlight 5.6).

Research Spotlight 5.6

Communication Training Enhances Empathy

In a study of communication education onsite in a veterinary practice, after training, veterinarians expressed significantly more emotional rapport statements, including expressions of empathy, reassurance, and legitimation (Shaw et al. 2016). As a result, it is important to recognize that empathy is a communication skill that can be developed with intention.

Partnership

Definition
Expressing the desire to work together toward a mutual goal. Clients at the veterinary clinic may feel overwhelmed, helpless, or as though they lack control, which may feel alienating or isolating. This is especially true when a client is highly concerned about their pet's well-being and uncertain about what is happening and may be asking themselves *What are the next steps?* or *What will this mean for my pet?*

Offering partnership relieves the pressure or burden, and clients no longer feel as though they are alone. Instead, the client perceives that a veterinary professional is by their side along the way. Research indicates that partnership is an underutilized skill in veterinarian–client interactions (Research Spotlight 5.7).

Research Spotlight 5.7

Lack of Partnership

In the detailed analysis of veterinarian–client–patient communication involving 150 preventive care and 150 health-related problem appointments, partnership statements were expressed in only 2% of appointments (Shaw et al. 2004). These results highlight the opportunity to incorporate partnership statements during interactions, to verbally convey support for our clients.

Technique

Use inclusive language to explicitly state the intention to work together and collaborate (Sidebar 5.4).

Sidebar 5.4   Partnership Language

> *Let's*
> *We*
> *Together*
> *Our*
> *Us*
> *As a team*
> *You and I*
> *You are not alone*
> *I would like to partner with you . . .*
> *I will be your guide through this . . .*
> *How can I help you?*
> *What support do you need from me?*

Examples

> **Let's** *take a moment to talk about your concerns about Chloe's urinary accidents.*
> **We** *will work* **together** *on a plan to address Chloe's accidents in a timely manner.*
> *How can* **I help you** *work through the various options?*

Asking Permission

Definition

Check to see if the other person is ready or will give consent to move forward in the conversation, procedure, agenda, or decision. Asking permission is both a relational skill, to obtain the other person's acceptance, and a structural skill, to assess the other person's readiness to take the next step. This skill was introduced in Chapter 4, as a considerate closed-ended inquiry to assess a client's readiness, and will be discussed again in Chapter 6, to respectfully phrase a signpost to transition the conversation; it is presented here as a skill that attends to relationships.

This simple act of respect gives clients or colleagues time to process options and ready themselves, be receptive to the message, and pace the conversation together. This skill puts the other person in the driver's seat, which is particularly helpful when broaching a difficult conversation or when a client feels helpless or out of control. If they are not ready to move forward, no matter how important the conversation, procedure, or decision may be, it is not productive or constructive to the relationship to proceed.

Technique

Propose a potential approach, procedure, conversation topic, or option, and stop to see if the client gives the go-ahead to move on to the topic or pursue the next step (Sidebar 5.5).

Sidebar 5.5   Asking Permission Stems

Would it be all right if . . .
I am wondering if . . .
What would it be like if . . .
Can we . . .
How would you feel if . . .
What do you think about . . .
Are you okay if . . .
Can I have your permission . . .
Would you mind if . . .
Might you consider . . .
Perhaps we could . . .
Are you ready to . . .

Examples

I am wondering if *we could talk some more about behavior modification for Chloe.*

Are you okay if *we now discuss diagnostic tests that may help us determine if there is a medical problem?*

Would you consider *consulting a veterinary behaviorist?*

Commonly Asked Questions About Attending to Relationships

What Is the Difference between Empathy and Reflective Listening?

Reflective listening and empathy are similar communication tools: both are important, and both help the client feel heard and understood (Morse et al. 2008). The difference is the content of the messages. With reflective listening, the content is often data-oriented or factual (*I heard you say that Chloe's behavior worsened when you were traveling more*). With empathy, the content is emotional, naming the feelings or experience of the other person (*It sounds like you are **concerned** that you may lose Chloe if she continues to have accidents outside of the litterbox*).

How Do I Use Self-Disclosure Effectively to Empathize with Others?

Self-disclosure is a form of empathy and a way to relate with another person. The challenge in self-sharing is ensuring that the focus stays on the client (Morse et al. 2008). To maintain attention on the client, keep the story's content short and redirect the conversation back to the client quickly. (*Our family felt conflicted about rehoming our cat, Tabatha. We were frustrated that she was peeing outside the litterbox. With support from a behaviorist to help us understand what was going on, we were able to resolve her behavioral issue. What has been your family's experience?*) Beware of relying on self-disclosure too often as a way of expressing empathy; consider developing other verbal expressions of empathy to form a connection.

How Do I Empathize without Getting Compassion Fatigue?

It is commonly perceived that keeping a safe emotional distance protects veterinary professionals from "compassion fatigue," a state of emotional and physical exhaustion and diminished ability to respond with empathy or compassion. However, we expend a lot of energy shielding ourselves from feelings, which is even more emotionally depleting. One of the greatest sources of fulfillment for us as veterinary professionals is time spent building relationships (Shaw et al. 2012).

Instead of a protective stance, try an open-hearted and self-loving approach. In empathizing with clients and patients, be open to receiving more than you give. Be present in the moment: it does not take much to offer words of understanding, be receptive to what clients share, and acknowledge their feelings. It is meaningful to share with clients in these intimate and compassionate moments.

It is draining to feel a need or responsibility to fix the problem. Without asking or being asked, we take the burden on ourselves, which may not be what the client is looking for. We then become resentful when we do too much for others. Often the client is only seeking to be heard, not fixed. Most people are asking only to be understood; and when they are, they often feel empowered to repair the situation themselves without our assistance.

What is often taken for granted is the need to direct the gift of empathy toward ourselves as well as to our clients and their pets. Self-kindness means treating ourselves as we would our clients, patients, and colleagues, with internal thoughts of understanding and support (Neff 2011). Rebalance through self-compassion as a protective buffer from the suffering of others.

Routine Client Scenario

Set the Scene: Dr. Howell sits down with Mr. Fitzgerald to talk through the steps in determining the cause of Chloe's inappropriate urination.

> ***This*** *inappropriate urination is a **stressful** situation for you and Chloe.* [empathy] *So,* ***would it be helpful to*** [asking permission] *walk through the steps of how* ***we*** [partnership] *might figure it out?*
> *The first step* ***we*** *can take **together** for Chloe* [partnership] *is to see if we can identify an underlying medical problem. This entails bloodwork and a urinalysis. We could proceed with that today **if you are willing**.* [asking permission]
> ***It sounds like*** *an **immediate** solution is needed, as your **family is fed up**.* [empathy]
> *It's important to identify or rule out a medical problem up front to best care for Chloe. Also, it may be easier and quicker for* ***us*** *to treat a medical problem over a behavior issue.* [partnership]
> *In the meantime,* ***let's*** *chat more about your household, stressors for Chloe, and litterbox hygiene to see if* ***we*** *can come up with some simple approaches.* [partnership]

Challenging Client Scenario

Set the Scene: Dr. Howell identifies a urinary tract infection, places Chloe on antibiotics, and schedules a two-week recheck examination. Two days later, a frustrated and disappointed Mr. Fitzgerald returns with Chloe for inappetence, vomiting, and diarrhea. Mr. Fitzgerald shares, *I thought we were out of the woods, and now Chloe's been vomiting and having diarrhea on our carpet.*

> *It sounds like Chloe is feeling terrible.* ***I can imagine*** *how **frustrating** it is for you to be cleaning up vomit and diarrhea, especially on top of the recent urinary accidents.* [empathy]
> *I'd like to* ***work with you*** *to get Chloe feeling better quickly.* [partnership]
> ***Can I share*** *with you what I think is going on?* [asking permission]
> *I fear that Chloe is reacting to the antibiotic for her urinary tract infection. I would like to propose that you leave her with us for the day, so we can rehydrate her, address her nausea, and look into another treatment option.* ***How would you feel about*** *leaving her with us?* [asking permission]
> ***I appreciate that*** *these side effects have been another **setback** for you and Chloe.* [empathy]
> ***I am confident that** **together we*** *will get her back on track shortly.* [partnership]

Talk Through Technology – Types of Communication

Consider how to align the type of communication with client preferences to enhance relationship-building. Many factors impact client comfort with technology, including familiarity, age, and access, so individualize the approach to meet each person's needs. This means eliciting client preferences, being flexible, and offering alternative options.

1. **Be flexible.** Keep communication preferences in mind. For instance, certain clients may be more comfortable with face-to-face, telephone, or email communication, while others may prefer video call, text, or social media. This means developing a level of comfort and competency with diverse modalities and meeting the needs of each individual client.

2. **Elicit preferences.** Ask clients the best way to communicate with them. *What is the best way to reach you? How would you like me to follow up with you? How would you like me to connect with you?*

3. **Offer options.** Clients may not be aware that they can schedule a virtual appointment, phone consultation, home, or in-person visit. It is stressful for clients and pets to go to the veterinary hospital. One option may work best to meet their special needs. For instance, not all clients can transport themselves and their pet to the clinic. Not all pets do well in the veterinary clinic setting. Coming to an appointment may require taking time off work, scheduling a babysitter, or sending a caregiver with the pet. When scheduling appointments, lay out the choices and ask the client what they prefer so they can determine what fits best for their lifestyle and their pet's personality. *What appointment type works best for you and your pet?*

4. **Use the appropriate modality.** Each type of communication serves a particular purpose. Take a minute to ask, *What is the most appropriate form of communication for this task?* For instance, delivering bad news is ideally conducted in person in a private setting (e.g. examination room). Confirming an appointment date and time is efficiently communicated in a reminder text. Negative test results can be shared in a text or email, whereas positive test results are best provided over the phone or in person to allow for discussion, questions, and clarification of next steps. A video call may be preferred over a telephone consultation to view and assess a patient.

Attend to Team Relationships

Making time to build relationships with colleagues is as important as doing so with clients. Team relationships form the foundation of practice culture. Colleague interactions impact team morale and job satisfaction and determine whether employees enjoy coming to work. Strong, trusting relationships at work promote loyalty and staff retention (Sidebar 5.6). Valuing people creates a workplace environment where colleagues jump in, are willing to help, provide support, and look after each other. This is critical to caring for others and managing the stress associated with the high-paced environment of a veterinary practice.

Sidebar 5.6   Team Outcomes of Attending to Relationships

Foster job satisfaction
Improve efficiency of interactions
Promote coordination of care
Support professional wellness
Enhance staff retention
Boost practice performance

Relationships within a veterinary team are built, maintained, and sustained using the same four communication skills identified earlier. Read the nonverbal signals of colleagues and check to see how they are doing and whether the interpretation was accurate. Checking in is a critical step, as it is easy to make assumptions or misinterpret the nonverbal cues of others, especially under pressure. Also, remain mindful of what is communicated through your nonverbal messages, and invite trusted colleagues to provide feedback and perceptions.

The opportunities to express empathy and offer partnership to colleagues are bountiful. Connect and relate to a colleague's life and work events, ranging from providing support and acknowledging hardship to celebrating accomplishments. Offer partnership to lend a hand and extend help. When we are not sure how to assist, we ask permission to see what our colleague may need or propose something to relieve their burden. Keep an eye out for opportunities to step in, and others will do the same in return.

Routine Team Scenario

Set the Scene: A patient in an emergency presents while Dr. Howell is discussing with Mr. Fitzgerald the diagnostic workup for Chloe. Fortunately, Dr. Howell is working with Julie, an experienced veterinary technician, and the two make a strong team.

> JULIE: *Can you triage the emergency patient?* [asking permission] *I can finish up the discharge with Mr. Fitzgerald and Chloe **for you**.* [partnership]
>
> DR. HOWELL: *Thanks, Julie! **Let's** reconvene and check back in **with each other** once the emergency case is evaluated and the patient's immediate needs are addressed.* [partnership]
>
> Julie attends to Mr. Fitzgerald and Chloe, discusses antibiotic administration, potential side effects, and the importance of a recheck examination and urinalysis, and assists Mr. Fitzgerald with checking out. Next, Julie returns to see how she can assist with the emergency patient.
>
> JULIE: *Mr. Fitzgerald and Chloe are on their way home. How are you doing? It's turned into a **crazy busy** morning for you.* [empathy]
>
> DR. HOWELL: *I need to hospitalize our emergency patient. **Would you mind** taking down the treatment plan?* [asking permission]
>
> JULIE: *Sure. How else can **I help you** right now?* [partnership]
>
> DR. HOWELL: *You did already! **I appreciate you** helping finish up and taking care of Mr. Fitzgerald and Chloe.* [partnership]

Challenging Team Scenario

Set the Scene: While Dr. Howell is writing up Chloe's medical record in the treatment room, Mari-Elena, another veterinary technician, approaches and states, *I can't believe you hospitalized that emergency patient when the clients didn't even have enough money to pay for the office visit.*

> DR. HOWELL: ***It sounds like** you're **concerned** about how they will pay their bill.* [empathy]
>
> MARI-ELENA: *I thought it was practice protocol that we don't hospitalize patients without a down payment on the treatment plan.*
>
> DR. HOWELL: ***May I share with you** what I learned from talking with these clients?* [asking permission]
>
> MARI-ELENA: *I guess, but you're not going to convince me otherwise.*
>
> DR. HOWELL: *I think **we** may see **eye to eye** on this once I share with you what is going on, as I know how passionate you are about animal welfare.* [partnership]

Put the Relationship Skills into Practice

Do-It-Yourself Exercises

Exercise 5.1   Skill Spot – Relational Skills
Review the following example phrases and label them as empathy, partnership, or asking-permission statements. The answer key is at the end of the chapter.

1. *I hope we can work together to find a swift solution.*

2. *Looks like you have a lot on your plate today. How can I help?*

3. *I can only imagine what a hassle it was to bring Chloe back in and to be cleaning up more messes in the house, not to mention your worry for Chloe.*

4. *Would you be willing to review this case with me? The patient is not responding to treatment so far, and I am concerned that I may have missed something.*

Exercise 5.2 Self-Assessment

Self-reflect on interactions with clients or colleagues. During the next few weeks practice the relational communication skills. After each appointment or collegial interaction, self-reflect using the following list of questions:

1. How familiar was I with this client or colleague?

2. What nonverbal cues did I see in my client or colleague? How did they contribute to the relationship?

3. What nonverbal behaviors did I sense in myself? What was their impact on the relationship?

4. How did I empathize with my client or colleague?

5. How did I offer partnership to my client or colleague?

6. How did I ask permission prior to proceeding?

7. How would I characterize the relationship at the end of the interaction?

Exercise 5.3 Next Steps for Success

1. Identify a coaching partner in the practice. Prioritize one of the four relationship communication skills (i.e. nonverbal behaviors, empathy, partnership, or asking permission) to work on. Inform your partner of your communication goal, invite them to observe one or more interactions, and request specific, balanced, descriptive and detailed feedback.

2. Be gentle and kind, as trying on a new communication skill is often awkward. It will take time and effort until it becomes automatic and authentic.

3. Repeat the cycle of honing in on one of the four relationship communication skills at a time, practicing, requesting feedback from a colleague, and self-assessing until you achieve competence with all four relationship communication skills.

Engage-the-Entire-Team Exercises

Exercise 5.4 Empathy Challenge

Challenge the team to begin a daily practice of expressing empathy with clients and colleagues:

1. Look for empathetic opportunities in client and colleague interactions.

2. Verbally express empathy in the moment.

3. Take note of the client's or colleague's response.

4. Record and capture the empathy statements on sticky notes, flip-chart paper, whiteboard, or posterboard in the treatment area to share with colleagues.

5. Designate time to present the poster in team meetings to celebrate strengths, reveal challenges, and share results of expressing empathy.

6. Over time, note changes in self, client, and colleague interactions and the practice culture.

Exercise 5.5   Find the Backstory

When the team feels more adept at expressing empathy, the next-level challenge is to highlight the results. Expressions of empathy often reveal more of the backstory behind the client's or colleague's emotions. When individuals feel acknowledged, it creates a safe place for them to be fully themselves and share more.

   The goal of this exercise is to use empathy to discover the backstory. Knowing the underlying story creates greater understanding and compassion for the client's or colleague's circumstances. What is it, exactly, that the client or colleague is going through?

1. Work in a small group of three individuals:
   a. One person reflects on an emotionally charged scenario that they would be willing to share with their colleagues.
   b. The second colleague invites the story and expresses verbal empathy in response at appropriate times.
   c. The third colleague observes and records the empathy examples, how the first individual responds, and what is learned.

2. After the role-play, debrief and reflect on the observed results:
   a. How did empathy move the interaction forward?
   b. How did the colleague sharing their emotionally charged scenario feel?
   c. What happened when the colleague's emotions were addressed?
   d. How did the colleague inviting the story feel?
   e. What new information was learned?
   f. What was the story behind the emotion?

Take It Away

1. Strike a balance between **building relationships and completing tasks** to build long-lasting connections and satisfying client and collegial relationships. This may entail slowing down initially to build rapport and then proceeding more quickly later in client or colleague interactions.
2. Pick up on **client or colleague nonverbal behaviors,** and reflect back what you see to check for accuracy.
3. Be aware of your **nonverbal behaviors** and how they are perceived by your clients and colleagues, and strive for congruency between nonverbal cues and verbal statements.
4. Sense your client's or colleague's emotions, and **express empathy** verbally to acknowledge and legitimize how they are feeling.
5. **Convey partnership** with clients and colleagues to work collaboratively toward common goals.
6. **Ask permission** to respectfully assess your client's or colleague's readiness to consider an approach, offer an idea, or take the next step.

Answer Key

Exercise 5.1 Skill Spot – Relational Skills

1. *I hope **we** can work **together** to find a swift solution.* [partnership]
2. *Looks like you have **a lot** on your plate today.* [empathy] *How can I **help**?* [partnership]
3. ***I can imagine** what a **hassle** it was to bring Chloe back in and to be cleaning up more messes in the house, not to mention your **worry** for Chloe.* [empathy]
4. ***Would you be willing to** review this case with me?* [asking permission] *The patient is not responding to treatment so far, and I am concerned that I may have missed something.*

References

Bylund, C.L. and Makoul, G. (2002). Empathetic communication and gender in the physician–patient encounter. *Patient Educ. Couns.* 48 (3): 207–216. https://doi.org/10.1016/S0738-3991(02)00173-8.

Carson, C. (2007). Nonverbal communication in veterinary practice. *Vet. Clin. Small Anim. Pract.* 37 (1): 49–63. https://doi.org/10.1016/j.cvsm.2006.10.001.

Coe, J.B., O'Connor, R.O., Pizzolon, C.N. et al. (2020). Investigation of the effects of veterinarians' attire on ratings of trust, confidence, and comfort in a sample of pet owners in Canada. *J. Am. Vet. Med. Assoc.* 256 (11): 1268–1276. https://doi.org/10.2460/javma.256.11.1268.

Cron, W.L., Slocum, J.V., Goonight, D.B., and Volk, J.O. (2000). Executive summary of the Brakke management and behavior study. *J. Am. Vet. Med. Assoc.* 217 (3): 332–338. https://doi.org/10.2460/javma.2000.217.332.

Hunter, L. and Shaw, J.R. (2012). Building a home to care for your clients: Part 1. *Exceptional Veterinary Team*. January/February: 14–18.

Kanji, N., Coe, J.B., Adams, C.L., and Shaw, J.R. (2012). Effect of veterinarian–client–patient interactions on client adherence to dentistry and surgery recommendations in companion-animal practice. *J. Am. Vet. Med. Assoc.* 240 (4): 427–436. https://doi.org/10.2460/javma.240.4.427.

McArthur, M.L. and Fitzgerald, J.R. (2013). Companion animal veterinarians' use of clinical communication skills. *Aust. Vet. J.* 91 (9): 374–380. https://doi.org/10.1111/avj.12083.

Mehrabian, A. (1972). *Nonverbal Communication*. Aldine-Atherton.

Mehrabian, A. (1971). *Silent Messages*. Wadsworth.

Morse, D.S., McDaniel, S.H., Candib, L.M., and Beach, M.C. (2008). "Enough about me, let's get back to you": physician self-disclosure during primary care encounters. *Ann. Intern. Med.* 149 (11): 835–837. https://doi.org/10.7326/0003-4819-149-11-200812020-00015.

Neff, K. (2011). *Self-Compassion: The Proven Power of Being Kind to Yourself*. New York, NY: Harper Publishers.

Shaw, J.R., Adams, C.L., Bonnett, B.N. et al. (2004). Use of the Roter interaction analysis system to analyze veterinarian–client–patient communication in companion animal practice. *J. Am. Vet. Med. Assoc.* 225 (2): 222–229. https://doi.org/10.2460/javma.2004.225.222.

Shaw, J.R., Adams, C.L., Bonnett, B.N. et al. (2008). Veterinarian–client–patient communication during wellness appointments versus appointments related to a health problem in companion animal practice. *J. Am. Vet. Med. Assoc.* 233 (10): 1576–1586. https://doi.org/10.2460/javma.233.10.1576.

Shaw, J.R., Barley, G.E., Hill, A.E. et al. (2010). Communication skills onsite in a veterinary practice. *Patient Educ. Couns.* 80 (3): 337–344. https://doi.org/10.1016/j.pec.2010.06.012.

Shaw, J.R., Adams, C.L., Bonnett, B.N. et al. (2012). Veterinarian satisfaction with companion animal visits. *J. Am. Vet. Med. Assoc.* 240 (7): 832–841. https://doi.org/10.2460/javma.240.7.832.

Shaw, J.R., Barley, G.E., Hill, A.E. et al. (2016). Outcomes assessment of onsite communication skills education in a companion animal practice. *J. Am. Vet. Med. Assoc.* 249 (4): 429–432. https://doi.org/10.2460/javma.249.4.419.

6

Attending to Tasks

Abstract

Attending to tasks is the organizational backbone that supports our client and collegial interactions. It provides the scaffolding for what is to happen next by providing necessary order for a complex process. Structured conversations reduce uncertainty, foster accuracy, and promote efficient problem-solving and decision-making. The relational skills set a tone of compassion and support, and the structural skills get the job done. Demonstrating compassion while efficiently attending to tasks is not easy; achieving both requires strong communication skills. The structural communication skills, introduced in this chapter, navigate the appointment roadmap in a timely manner; they allow us to take the lead and gently steer the conversation forward to ensure that goals are met and we arrive at the destination together. When the discussion gets off track, the tools guide the interaction back on course. In this chapter, we explore three communication skills for attending to tasks with clients or colleagues: logical sequence, signpost, and internal summary.

SELF-ASSESSMENT QUESTIONS

1. How do I establish structure at the outset of an appointment or meeting?
2. How do I transition between parts of an appointment or meeting?
3. How do I redirect when the appointment or meeting goes off course?

Introduction

The previous chapter focused on relational skills, as trust and rapport are at the heart of connections with clients and colleagues. Attending to tasks is the organizational backbone that supports interactions. It provides the scaffolding for what is to happen next by providing necessary order for a complex process. Structured conversations reduce uncertainty, foster accuracy, and promote efficient problem-solving and decision-making. The relational skills set a tone of compassion and support, and the structural or task-oriented skills get the job done. (Sidebar 6.1).

Sidebar 6.1   A Balancing Act between Relationship and Task

Relational Goals

Establish rapport
Provide support
Encourage participation
Empower roles
Invite contributions

Task Goals

Negotiate agendas
Meet deadlines
Address expectations
Fulfill responsibilities

Although powerful together, in a veterinary practice, relational and structural skill sets are often viewed as opposing each other, which is a daily source of tension and stress. We try to connect with the client and care for the patient while maintaining the appointment, treatment, and surgery schedules. Demonstrating compassion while efficiently attending to tasks is not easy; achieving both requires strong communication skills.

The most frequently expressed concern about relationship building is **I don't have time** or **The client goes on forever** about unrelated tangential topics. When communication goes astray, the structural skills respectfully get the conversation back on track to achieve critical outcomes of appointment flow and efficiency, reduce client uncertainty, and engender client confidence (Sidebar 6.2).

Sidebar 6.2   Clinical Outcomes of Attending to Tasks

Create flow
Enhance efficiency
Reduce uncertainty
Engender confidence

The structure of the clinical interview forms the outline for the appointment (Figure 6.1). To start, attend to tasks with a clear organizational structure for the appointment: opening-the-interaction, information-gathering, physical examination, diagnostic and treatment planning, and closing-the-interaction. This is the big-picture framework of the interaction in our mind going into the visit. We share these steps with our client by explicitly stating where we are going. And before moving on, we check and see if it is all right to proceed or if our client might like to pursue a different path based on their priorities.

Second, we establish common goals and a shared vision for moving forward by eliciting a mutual agenda. As described in Chapter 3, we elicit our client's or our colleague's agenda and put forth our items to establish a joint agenda. With the list in hand, we begin with the end in mind. After exploring each party's ideas, lay out a proposed route of concerns, topics, or issues to address that keeps everyone traveling on the same path. We refer to the roadmap throughout the interaction to ensure that all parties' goals, expectations, and priorities are met along the way, and we arrive at the destination together in a timely manner.

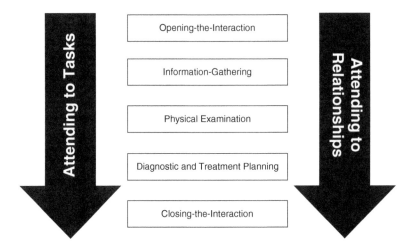

Figure 6.1 Structure of the clinical interview. *Source:* Skills for Communicating with Patients, 3rd Edition by Silverman J, Kurtz S, Draper J. Copyright 2013 by Imprint. Reproduced by permission of Taylor and Francis Group.

Finally, we use the attending-to-tasks communication skills to navigate the roadmap during the appointment; they allow us to take the lead and gently guide the conversation forward. When the discussion gets off track, the skills steer the interaction back within established boundaries. Throughout the conversation, we are cognizant of whether our client is tracking with us by regularly assessing if they are ready to move on to the next topic; and if not, we loop back to bring them with us. This process helps the veterinary team stay the course even when running behind, triaging emergencies, and juggling other time-intensive demands. In this chapter, we explore three communication skills for attending to tasks with clients or colleagues: logical sequence, signpost, and internal summary (Sidebar 6.3). We provide examples in two settings: in the examination room, working with Mrs. Chavez and Penelope; and during a team meeting led by the practice manager, Nguyen.

Sidebar 6.3 Communication Skills for Attending to Tasks

Logical sequence
Signpost
Internal summary

Set the Scene

Client Scenario: Mrs. Chavez is a long-time client who presents with Penelope, a six-year-old female-spayed Pomeranian, to see Dr. Suarez for acute diarrhea of two days' duration. Mrs. Chavez is tired of cleaning up all the messes in the house and is concerned that Penelope is getting dehydrated. Penelope's diet was changed recently, and the family is hosting out-of-town guests, who are giving Penelope more treats to coax her out of hiding. On top of it all, Mrs. Chavez is planning her daughter's wedding and hosting the bridal shower this weekend.

Team Scenario: A team meeting led by the practice manager, Nguyen, is just starting with three agenda items: reviewing client feedback, providing an update on compensation and benefits package, and setting a date for the clinic's annual summer barbecue. The compensation and benefits discussion will likely bleed into the next team meeting.

Stepping into Dr. Suarez's and Nguyen's shoes, self-reflect on:

1. How would I help Mrs. Chavez focus on Penelope instead of wedding plans?
2. How would I facilitate a collaborative and productive team discussion to address all three topics within the allotted meeting time?

Attend to Client Tasks

Key Communication Skills for Attending to Tasks

The process or **how** of attending to tasks is the way we use key communication skills to structure, redirect, and stay on track in the conversation.

Logical Sequence

Definition
Structuring an appointment using a natural flow and progression from opening-the-interaction, including agenda-setting, to information-gathering, performing a physical examination, discussing diagnostic and treatment plans, and closing-the-interaction.

Technique
Take a logical and systematic approach from the opening to the closing of the appointment (Sidebar 6.4). Complete each step before progressing to the next, and be mindful of jumping ahead or moving too quickly.

> **Sidebar 6.4 Logical Sequence of the Clinical Interview**
>
> Opening-the-interaction
> Information-gathering
> Physical examination
> Diagnostic and treatment planning
> Closing-the-interaction

Getting ahead, lingering behind, or detouring from the structure of the appointment leads to struggles with time management, diagnostic accuracy, and patient care. Following a methodological process safeguards against taking shortcuts or skipping critical steps in conducting a full patient assessment and proceeding through the clinical reasoning process. Stick to the structure to maintain a rigorous and robust diagnostic process.

To illustrate, if we leapfrog over agenda-setting to information-gathering, we might not hear the client's goals for the appointment, possibly leading to an "oh, by the way" moment at the end of the interaction (Dysart et al. 2011). If we develop a management plan without a comprehensive history, there may be significant gaps in our clinical reasoning, leading to backtracking with the client or, worse, misdiagnosis. Similarly, bouncing between information-gathering and diagnostic and treatment planning increases the likelihood of missing a key piece of historical data or physical examination finding, potentially leading to a medical error. So, we can use logical sequencing to guide ourselves and the client stepwise through the appointment.

Even if we outline a logical progression for the appointment, the client may take the conversation in an unexpected direction. The advantage of a prepared roadmap is to transition our way back when the conversation strays. We need to be flexible and remain open to informative and productive detours. This requires making course corrections in the moment and adjusting to meet the needs of our client and ourselves.

Signpost

Definition

A transitional statement that signals where the conversation has been and/or where it is going next by outlining a new direction for the discussion or by signaling a change in topic. Signposting is also used to emphasize an important point in the discussion. A "warning shot" is a specialized signpost used specifically to deliver bad news. It warns the client of challenging, surprising, or stressful information and allows them to prepare and ready themselves and rally their coping skills. For example, *I have unexpected findings to share with you* or *This is difficult news for me to share and for you to hear.*

Technique

Provide verbal direction to the conversation that bridges or transitions from one topic to the next, highlights important points for the client to remember, or offers a warning in advance of a difficult discussion. The skill of asking permission, presented in Chapter 5, is a form of signposting. It is a respectful and gentle way of asking a client if they are ready to segue into the next topic, proceed with a transaction, approve a procedure, or discuss a sensitive topic. Sidebar 6.5 lists examples of stems for formulating a signpost statement.

> ### Sidebar 6.5 Signpost Stems
>
> *Let's next . . .*
> *Now I'd like to . . .*
> *The next step . . .*
> *This is a critical point to remember . . .*
> *Here's another thought . . .*
> *Importantly . . .*
> *Can we start with . . .*
> *Before we talk about that, can we discuss . . .*
> *There are three options. The first is . . .*
> *The advantage of this approach is . . .*

Examples

> *Thank you. I have a good sense of the diarrhea,* **so now let's talk about** *the changes to Penelope's diet.* [topic transition]
> **It is important** *that if the diarrhea persists, you bring Penelope back immediately to prevent further dehydration.* [important point]
> **This is what I am worried about.** [warning shot] *With receiving more treats, I am concerned that she may have over-indulged.*

When clients get lost during the veterinary consultation, they become confused and stressed. It is important to notice when we lose them and provide explicit direction to get them back on track. Reducing uncertainty by setting expectations, laying out a plan, and taking a step-by-step approach – signposting – diffuses emotions and puts an anxious client at ease (Stoewen et al. 2019). Make structure explicit – even if it feels too planned, organized, or forced – by outlining the discussion. We can use signposting to guide ourselves and the client stepwise through the appointment (Box 6.1).

Box 6.1   During the Appointment, Use Signposting To . . .

1. Transition from the opening to agenda-setting.

   It is nice to meet you! ***I'd like to start our visit by*** *getting a clear picture of what we can do for you and Penelope today.*

2. Bridge from agenda-setting to information-gathering.

   Now that we have a plan for today's visit, *would you mind sharing with me what's been going on with Penelope?*

3. Shift from one topic to the next.

   So, it started with diarrhea. *Now, I'd like to ask you about what other changes you noticed?*

4. Switch between the current problems to past medical history.

   I know Penelope is here for diarrhea. *To ensure that I'm not missing something,* ***I want to explore her past medical problems***.

5. Start the physical exam.

   Would it be all right if I examined Penelope now *to see what might be going on?*

6. Discuss diagnostic and treatment planning.

   Let's talk about *some things we can do to make Penelope feel better.*

7. Delineate the diagnostic options.

   There are ***two paths*** *we can take moving forward:*
   - *We can run blood and poop tests to identify an underlying cause.*
   - *Or we can treat the diarrhea to see how Penelope responds.*

8. Preface treatment options.

   There are ***three supportive treatments*** *to help Penelope feel better:*
   - *The* ***first*** *is putting fluids under her skin to treat her dehydration.*
   - ***Meanwhile***, *feed her a bland diet that is gentle on her stomach.*
   - *And* ***finally***, *we'll administer a probiotic to get her back on track.*

9. Outline the advantages and disadvantages of each option.

   The ***disadvantage*** *of the supportive care path is that we don't know the underlying cause. If* ***Penelope's diarrhea persists***, *we'll need to hospitalize her, run tests, and treat aggressively then.*

10. Prepare to close the interview.

    Let's wrap up *our appointment.*

11. Highlight important points.

    There are a ***couple of key points*** *to keep in mind. If Penelope does not improve overnight, I'd like to see her again first thing in the morning. If the diarrhea continues, she is at risk of becoming dehydrated and will require hospitalization and intravenous fluids.*

Adapted from Hunter and Shaw (2011).

Signposting is one of the least intuitive and most difficult of the communication skills. It is not commonly used in social conversations. For professional dialogue, however, it is invaluable. Although the structure may be clear in our heads, it may not be so for our clients. And when, as veterinary professionals, we are confused about how to proceed, stating where we have been and where we are going (i.e. signposting) sometimes determines the next step forward.

Internal Summary

Definition

Reflecting a list of two or more items in order to demonstrate attentive listening; check for completeness, understanding, or accuracy; or invite further contributions. In this book, we introduce two types of summaries: internal summary was briefly introduced in Chapter 4 as a tool for pulling together data during information-gathering; and here, internal summary is covered in depth as a structural communication skill to be used in various places within the body of the appointment. In Chapter 8, end summary is discussed as a closing communication skill to conclude the visit.

Technique

Internal summaries are composed of two steps. The first is to review out loud the list of agenda items, information gathered, or diagnostic tests or treatment approaches available. The second is to check for accuracy and completeness to ensure that we did not miss items and the information is thorough. Sidebar 6.6 provides examples of stems to begin a summary statement. The same phrasing is used for both internal and end summary statements.

Sidebar 6.6   Summary Stems

To recap . . .
To summarize . . .
To pull it all together . . .
To make sure I have it all . . .
Let me see if I am correct . . .
Let me see if I got this right . . .
What I heard is . . .
What you are saying is . . .

Examples

Mrs. Chavez, **to summarize**, *you've noticed that Penelope had multiple bouts of watery diarrhea over the past two days. You changed her diet recently and are currently hosting houseguests who've been giving Penelope more treats. The good news is that Penelope's attitude, appetite, and energy level remain good.* [internal summary] **What** *else do you think I need to know?* [open-ended inquiry]
We decided to *provide supportive care for Penelope's diarrhea, including fluids under her skin, starting her on a bland diet, and giving her a probiotic.* [internal summary] *If Penelope's diarrhea persists,* [signpost] *we need to run blood tests and analyze her poop to look for something more serious.* **What** *questions do you have?* [open-ended inquiry]

Internal summary presents a mental rest stop for the client and veterinary professional to pull together data, take stock of what has been learned so far, and engage in the clinical reasoning process. When we summarize, we integrate and synthesize data on the fly. This is the skill we use to itemize, organize, and prioritize the clues to the case, form a diagnostic plan, or discover missing information. We identify gaps, inconsistencies, or contradictions that warrant further exploration or clarification.

Internal summaries are the perfect skill to make a recovery when we lose our train of thought or are not quite sure what to say or do next. It also serves as a checkpoint to ensure that the client feels heard. There are multiple places to summarize throughout the appointment (Box 6.2).

Box 6.2 Opportunities to Summarize During the Appointment

1. Reflect what you recall from previous visits:

   I read in the notes that *Penelope is up to date on her preventive care, and her past visits were only for annual examinations. What did I miss?*

2. Share what you learned from the veterinary technician:

   My veterinary technician, Tory, shared with me that *Penelope has had diarrhea for the past two days. Despite that, she is acting like her normal self. What else would you like to share?*

3. Capture the client's full agenda:

   On our list for today is *investigating the diarrhea. Your goal is to make it stop, as you're concerned that Penelope may be getting dehydrated. What else would you like to discuss?*

4. Outline data-gathered:

   So, it sounds like *the potential culprits are the change in diet, houseguests, and getting more treats. What else may be contributing?*

5. Present physical examination findings:

   On Penelope's physical exam, *she is showing signs of mild dehydration and a sensitive belly on palpation. All else checks out normal. What can I clarify?*

6. Explain what we will learn from diagnostic tests:

   So, ***if we run bloodwork and the poop test****, we may find an underlying cause for Penelope's diarrhea, so we'll know how to target her treatment. What are your thoughts?*

7. Highlight advantages and disadvantages of each treatment option:

   To summarize, the downside *to treating first and watching for her response is that if Penelope's diarrhea persists, I am concerned she will get severely dehydrated. How would you like to proceed?*

8. Close the visit:

   You brought Penelope in for *diarrhea over the past two days. You recently changed her diet, and she is getting extra treats from houseguests. On her examination, she is slightly dehydrated with a sensitive belly. We decided to start with supportive care, including fluids under the skin, feeding a bland diet, and taking a probiotic. What questions do you have?*

Commonly Asked Questions About Attending to Tasks

How Do I Rein in Clients Who Go Off on Tangents?

An initial consideration in addressing this question is realizing that our impression about how long clients speak is often inaccurate. In one seminal communication study, patients in human medicine were found to take no more than 150 seconds to complete their statement of concerns (Beckman and Frankel 1984). A similar study in veterinary medicine reported that clients took no more than 139 seconds to share their concerns (Dysart et al. 2011). So, take a breath, as clients are often not "going on and on" as long as we think.

Next, reflect on what client's perspective or environmental content is truly tangential in nature. Our clients' stories often contain important clues to the diagnosis or barriers to their ability to care for their pets that we may not otherwise discover. This information may inadvertently contribute to our clinical reasoning, diagnostic accuracy, or client adherence. If we try to corral the conversation too heavy-handedly, we may miss it.

If the client says something truly tangential, agenda-setting (Chapter 3) serves as a contract. If the topic is off agenda, redirect back to the concerns at hand using a signpost, such as *I know we agreed that it is important that we talk about . . .*, or listen carefully in case the client is raising a late-arising agenda item – *It sounds like we need to add that to today's agenda for discussion.*

Routine Client Scenario

Set the Scene: When Dr. Suarez walks into the examination room, Mrs. Chavez excitedly begins to share.

> **MRS. CHAVEZ:**   *It is finally happening! I'm planning my daughter's wedding! I've been busy – shopping for a bridal gown and bridesmaid dresses, scheduling wedding cake tastings, sending out the last of the wedding invitations, and finalizing the menu with the caterer. The price of the wedding planner was worth it! This weekend is the bridal shower. Our relatives started arriving a couple of days ago. They're staying at the house, and of all times, Penelope has terrible watery diarrhea.*
>
> **DR. SUAREZ:**   ***Sounds like** an exciting time, and a full household.* [reflective listening] *Thanks for bringing Penelope in. Before we dive in, **can I outline** today's visit for us?* [signpost – asking permission]
> ***I'd like to learn** more about what has been going on with you and Penelope in general. **Then** we'll focus on her horrible diarrhea problem, examine Penelope, and **come up with a plan** to get her feeling better.* [logical sequence] ***How** does that sound to you?* [open-ended inquiry]
> *Given how **busy** things sound,* [empathy] ***would you be okay if we** move on to discussing Penelope's diarrhea?* [signpost – asking permission]
> ***Let's start with** what the diarrhea looks like.* [signpost] ***Would that be okay?*** [asking permission]

Challenging Client Scenario

Set the Scene: The conversation in the examination room continues.

> **MRS. CHAVEZ:**   *Did I tell you that my relatives have taken over the house? Penelope is spending a lot of time hiding in her cave under my bed. Poor thing! In trying to befriend her, the guests have been trying to coax her out from under the bed with lots of treats.*
>
> **DR. SUAREZ:**   *Mrs. Chavez, **I heard you mention** several times now how much is going on for you with your daughter's bridal shower and that it's an exciting time, which has also been*

stressful. It has also been anxiety-producing for Penelope and you are wondering whether the stress may be causing her diarrhea. [internal summary] ***What*** *else would you like to add?* [open-ended inquiry]

MRS. CHAVEZ: *Yeah, Penelope doesn't like company. She is not coping well with all the houseguests, which I think maybe causing the diarrhea.*

DR. SUAREZ: *That's certainly possible. I've got a* ***few more questions****, and* ***after that*** *I'd like to do a thorough physical examination.* [signpost] ***How*** *does that sound to you?* [open-ended inquiry]

Let's talk about *stress-reduction techniques for Penelope* [signpost] *in addition to treating her diarrhea. It sounds like they may go together.*

Talk Through Technology – Virtual Care

A virtual visit is an effective method to serve clients and patients at a distance when they cannot attend an appointment in person. Such interactions may occur over the phone, via a video call, or virtual platform. What is common to all forms of virtual care is the loss of nonverbal communication, making it even more important to be intentional with our verbal communication skills. Here are some recommendations to set expectations, reduce uncertainty, and stay on track:

1. **Orient the client to the visit.** Make an introduction, include your name and clarify your role, take a minute to perform a technology check-in to be sure the video and/or sound are working appropriately and the client can hear, and then orient the client to how the appointment will proceed (Box 6.3).

Box 6.3   Structuring a Virtual Appointment

Set the Scene: Given her busy schedule, Mrs. Chavez requested a virtual follow-up appointment for Penelope. She did not have the time for an in-person veterinary visit because of wedding planning.

> *Hello Mrs. Chavez, I'm Janna, one of the veterinary technicians,* [make introduction to the client and clarify your role] *and I am caring for you and Penelope today.* ***Before we proceed,*** [signpost] *can you hear and see me all right? Please let me know if you have technological difficulties at any point, and* ***I will help you.*** [partnership]
> ***I'm wondering*** *what your experience is with virtual appointments.* [open-ended inquiry] ***If it's all right with you****, let me explain how it works.* [signpost – asking permission] ***First*** *I will ask you some initial questions about Penelope, and* ***then*** *Dr. Suarez will follow up, likely with more questions.* ***Next,*** *with your help, we will examine Penelope.* ***Finally****, Dr. Suarez will provide an update and discuss recommendations for further examination, tests, or treatments for Penelope – if needed [signpost – logical sequence].* ***What*** *questions do you have?* [open-ended inquiry]

---

2. **Elicit the client's agenda.** Since the client is not onsite to advocate for their expectations, it is of utmost importance to identify upfront the reasons for the visit, including the client's concerns, goals, expectations, and priorities for the visit. Summarize what the client shared, and check to see if there are other agenda items (as discussed in Chapter 3).

3. **Maintain the logical sequence of a traditional appointment.** In feeling literally distant from the veterinary practice and team, clients may come to a virtual appointment with anxiety.

Stick to the familiar structure of the clinical interview to assure clients receive the same level of quality care for their pet and customer service for themselves.

4. **Ask permission to transition.** Signpost to indicate the next step or topic in the virtual interaction. Without our client's nonverbal cues, we may advance before the client is ready to do so. They may need more time to process information or to pose additional questions. Asking permission creates a checkpoint for the client to indicate if or when we can progress with the appointment. This minimizes the chances of losing the client along the way or causing discomfort and nervousness with a new format for a veterinary visit.

5. **Summarize at regular intervals.** Provide internal summaries throughout the virtual interaction by tracking the details for the client and yourself. This step ensures accurate and complete transfer of information and allows the client to feel heard. Summarize the key historical data gathered, highlight diagnostic or treatment steps, and summarize again at the end of the visit to ensure that everyone is on the same page.

6. **Integrate visual aids.** Depending on the platform, consider using the chat window, notes function, share screen, or whiteboard to visually present or capture specifics. Send handouts, pictures, websites, or charts to clients via email beforehand. In following up, send a care plan to the client with written instructions for how to treat their pet at home. Clients can refer to these documents later to address questions or provide clarification.

7. **Pause often.** Without nonverbal cues, it is easy to interrupt our clients during virtual visits. Allow for even longer pauses than normal (six seconds versus three) to take turns speaking. This provides a break to take a breath and for the client to process what's been said and reflect on the next step.

8. **Lean on verbal relationship skills.** Especially with new client relationships, connection can be lost during virtual visits. What is missed with the lack of nonverbal communication is made up for with relational skills, such as expressing verbal empathy and offering partnership.

9. **Use available nonverbal communication.** On the phone, use vocal tone, pace, volume, and pitch to send the right message. On a video call, use eye contact, body position, facial expressions, leaning in, and head nodding to relate to and engage with the client.

Attend to Team Tasks

Even more so than with client interactions, in the day to day demands of veterinary practice, relational and structural skills often appear at odds with each other. We try to balance teamwork, collaboration, and morale-building as well as meet deadlines, fulfill the expectations and obligations of our roles, and responsibly complete our daily tasks. Some days we favor attending to tasks to get the work done, other days we are more focused on relationships and caring for the team, and then there are days when we strike the perfect balance! When the team is humming along, the day flows efficiently, expectations are clearly outlined, and decision-making is a seamless process (Sidebar 6.7).

Sidebar 6.7   Team Outcomes of Attending to tasks

Create flow
Enhance efficiency
Set expectations
Reduce uncertainty
Foster the decision-making process

The structural communication skills that keep veterinary professionals and clients on the same page are equally helpful in navigating colleague and team interactions. Following a logical structure applies to both team meetings and one-on-one collegial interactions. Start with an opening followed by setting a mutual agenda, information-gathering, identifying "action" items, and closing-the-meeting (Figure 6.2).

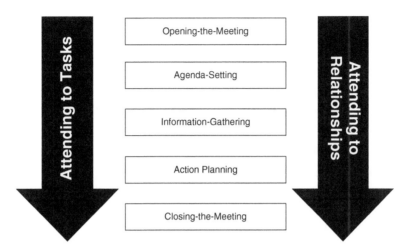

Figure 6.2   Structure of the team meeting. Adapted from Silverman et al. 2013 with permission.

During meetings, signposting acts like a GPS (i.e., global positioning system) (Box 6.4). This is how we provide direction to a colleague or team about what will be discussed, indicate where the meeting is heading next, and flag next steps for follow-through. Doing so ensures efficient, focused, and productive team meetings so the veterinary team remains engaged and on track.

Box 6.4   During a Meeting, Use Signposting To . . .

1. Support agenda-setting.

   I shared the meeting agenda. *What would you like to add?*

2. Introduce the first agenda item.

   Shall we start with *the first thing on our list?*

3. Progress to the next agenda item.

   What else would you like to share **before we move on to the next item**?

4. List information, options, or solutions.

   I have **three updates** *that I'd like to share with you.*
   We've come up with **two potential** *solutions.*
   We can approach this in **several ways.** *What might be most effective to start with?*

5. Transition to summarizing the action items generated.

   So, **before we close, let's go over our list of next steps**.

6. Inform the team about the next meeting.

   Our next meeting *is scheduled for Monday at 3:00 p.m.*

For team communication, internal summary is likewise an instrumental skill for pulling together everyone's ideas so they feel heard and valued for their contributions. Internal summary also checks for accuracy and thoroughness to ensure that we did not miss items and the information gathered is complete. There are multiple places during a meeting when internal summary puts critical pieces in place (Box 6.5).

Box 6.5   Opportunities to Summarize during a Meeting

1. Review the new agenda items submitted:

   So, on today's agenda *is reviewing next month's schedule; implementing an onboarding plan for Allison, our new veterinary technician; and budgeting for anticipated equipment purchases in the coming year. What else is on your minds?*

2. Highlight key points for discussion on a topic:

   The challenges for this month's *schedule are summer vacations, rotating Allison in at the end of the month, and accounting for one doctor who is away on parental leave. What else do we need to plan for?*

3. Recap action items that arise during the meeting:

   To onboard Allison*, Maria is going to put together an orientation checklist, Allison will job-shadow April for the first week, and I will update the policies and procedures manual. How else can we set Allison up for success?*

4. Review all the action items at the end of the meeting:

   Here's what I have*: Jamal is going to draw up a schedule for approval, Maria is putting together an orientation checklist, we have a team in place for mentoring Allison, and I will draft a budget proposal for equipment purchases for review. What am I missing?*

5. Outline items for discussion at the next meeting:

   On our list for Monday's meeting is *to review client survey feedback results, update team compensation and benefits package, and set a date for our annual summer barbecue. What else is on your radar?*

Routine Team Scenario

Set the Scene: It is the start of the team meeting, led by the practice manager, Nguyen.

> ***Let's look at*** *today's agenda together.* [signpost] *On our **discussion list** is recent client feedback. We'd like to identify what is working well, as well as opportunities for growth. We also wanted to update our compensation and benefits package and set dates for our annual barbecue.* [internal summary] ***What*** *else would you like to discuss today?* [open-ended inquiry]
>
> ***Are you okay if*** *we place team building on next week's agenda, when we'll have more time to address it fully?* [signpost – asking permission]
>
> ***Let's start with*** *recent client feedback.* [signpost]
>
> ***It sounds like*** *appointment wait times were the key issue in client feedback.* ***We discussed*** *informing clients ahead of time if we are running behind, offering to reschedule, sending in a client service coordinator or veterinary technician to get the appointment started, and offering*

an apology, update, and refreshments. [internal summary] **What** *else would you include?* [open-ended inquiry]

The next item, [signpost] *compensation and benefits package, may require more time. Perhaps* **we can start** *by brainstorming today.* [signpost]

Let's go back to *the previous item,* [signpost] *client feedback, as more ideas are still coming to the forefront.*

So, *given the amount of discussion and the fact that we are* **approaching the end of the meeting,** *[signpost]* **would you be comfortable** *continuing our conversation on compensation and benefits package at next week's meeting?* [signpost – asking permission]

Before we wrap up, [signpost] *let's look at our calendars to set a date for the summer barbecue.*

At our next meeting, [signpost] *let's pick up where we left off with compensation and benefits package. We also want to discuss team building as a new topic.* [internal summary] **What** *have I missed?* [open-ended inquiry]

Challenging Team Scenario

Set the Scene: During the follow-up meeting, the team is brainstorming ideas for team building. Nguyen is facilitating the meeting. A two-sided conversation erupts, and team members interrupt and speak over each other.

> MARIANA ASKS JONATHON: *What about initiating team huddles at the beginning of the day to celebrate accomplishments and identify needs and support for the day ahead?* **Simultaneously,** BARBARA ASKS SAUL *What if we read positive client reviews to start each day?*
>
> NGUYEN: *I'm sorry. I'm struggling to follow all the conversations.* **Let's back up a minute.** [signpost]
>
> **I've heard** *several good ideas, and I want to ensure that we capture them all.* [signpost] **Would you mind** *repeating them one at a time,* **starting with Mariana**? [signpost – asking permission]
>
> **So,** *we can add two more team-building items to our list: team huddles and sharing positive reviews at the start of the day.* [internal summary] **What** *other approaches might we consider?* [open-ended inquiry]
>
> **We still have 10 minutes** *remaining to finish brainstorming.* [signpost] **What** *other suggestions do you have?* [open-ended inquiry]

Put the Task Skills into Practice

Do-It-Yourself Exercises

Exercise 6.1   Skill Spot – Signposts and Internal Summaries

Review the following example phrases and label them as signpost or internal summary statements. The answer key is at the end of the chapter.

1. *Let's start by talking about how the diarrhea started.*

2. *You shared with me that this is a stressful time for you and Penelope, with your daughter's wedding. The last thing you need is a sick dog on top of a houseful of guests. It seems like the diarrhea*

may be stress-related, although the change in diet and eating more treats may also have contributed.

3. *We will open our next meeting with a discussion of compensation and benefits package.*

4. *It is important that if the diarrhea persists, we need to hospitalize Penelope to treat her dehydration.*

5. *In our previous meeting, we discussed recent client feedback and chose the date for our summer barbeque, and tabled compensation and benefits package and team-building for today's topics.*

Exercise 6.2   Client Communication Plan

Use the following prompts to outline a structural roadmap for an upcoming preventive care appointment. This is an exercise in explicitly stating the structure of transitioning from one section to the next. This map serves as a guide for where to go next, preventing runaway agendas and keeping appointments on time. The challenge is staying open to the client's agenda, sharp turns, and detours despite a structured plan. Be prepared to adapt the outline based on the client's agenda, and be open to new items or questions that may arise.

Write a signpost to support the following transitions:

1. Opening-the-interaction to agenda-setting

2. Agenda-setting to information-gathering

3. Information-gathering to physical examination

4. Physical examination to diagnostic and treatment planning

5. Diagnostic and treatment planning to closing-the-interaction

Exercise 6.3   Team Communication Plan

Using the same approach, create a conversational roadmap for a topic(s) you plan to raise during an upcoming team meeting. This map outlines where to go next, ensures that the team is working on the same agenda, and keeps meetings on track. The structural skills aid time management which is challenging when addressing a full meeting agenda.

Write a signpost to support the following transitions:

1. Opening-the-meeting to reviewing the agenda (i.e. topic(s) to address)

2. Agenda-setting to information-gathering

3. Information-gathering to formulating action plans

4. Action planning to closing-the-meeting

Exercise 6.4   Next Steps for Success

1. Based on what you learned from this chapter and the previous exercises, identify opportunities for growth by prioritizing one of the three attending-to-tasks communication skills (i.e. logical structure, signpost, or internal summary) to focus on for a solid week.

2. Identify a coaching partner in the practice familiar with the three structural communication skills. Inform them of your communication goal, invite them to observe an interaction, and request specific, descriptive, balanced, and relevant feedback.

3. Be gentle and kind, as trying on a new communication skill is often awkward. It will take time and effort until it becomes automatic and authentic.

4. Repeat the cycle of honing in on one communication skill, practicing, requesting feedback from a colleague, and self-assessment until you achieve competence with all three.

Take It Away

1. Guide the client through the **logical sequence** of the clinical appointment or the veterinary team through a team meeting.
2. **Signpost** frequently along the way to guide the conversation and keep clients and colleagues on track.
3. **Summarize** during appointments to confirm facts, pull data together, integrate clinical reasoning, and stay side by side. Summarize during meetings to keep track of key ideas, action items, and plans for moving forward.

Answer Key

Exercise 6.1   Skill Spot – Signposts and Internal Summaries
1. *Let's start by* talking about how the diarrhea started. [signpost]
2. *You shared with me that* this is a stressful time for you and Penelope, with your daughter's wedding. The last thing you need is a sick dog on top of a houseful of guests. It seems like the diarrhea may be stress-related, although the change in diet and eating more treats may also have contributed. [internal summary]
3. *We will open our next meeting with* a discussion of compensation and benefits package. [signpost]
4. *It is important that if the diarrhea persists*, we need to hospitalize Penelope to treat her dehydration. [signpost]
5. *In our previous meeting, we discussed* recent client feedback and chose the date for our summer barbeque, and tabled compensation and benefits package and team-building for today's topics. [internal summary]

References

Beckman, H.B. and Frankel, R.M. (1984). The effect of physician behavior on the collection of patient data. *Ann. Intern. Med.* 101 (5): 692–696. https://doi.org/10.7326/0003-4819-101-5-692.

Dysart, L.M., Coe, J.B., and Adams, C.L. (2011). Analysis of solicitation of client concerns in companion animal practice. *J. Am. Vet. Med. Assoc.* 238 (12): 1609–1615. https://doi.org/10.2460/javma.238.12.1609.

Hunter, L. and Shaw, J.R. (2011). Are We There Yet? *Veterinary Team Brief*. November/December: 4–7.

Riccardi, V.M. and Kurtz, S.M. (1983). *Communication and Counseling in Health Care*. Springfield, IL: Charles C. Thomas Publisher.

Silverman, J., Kurtz, S., and Draper, J. (2013). *Skills for Communicating with Patients*. London, England. CRC Press.

Stoewen, D.L., Coe, J.B., MacMartin, C., Stone, E.A., and Dewey, C.E. (2019). Identification of Illness uncertainty in veterinary oncology: implications for service. *Front. Vet. Sci.* 6: 147. https://doi.org/10.3389/fvets.2019.00147.

7

Diagnostic and Treatment Planning

Abstract

Diagnostic and treatment planning conversations are the most complex of the clinical interview. What is learned during agenda-setting and information-gathering serves as the foundation on which to build a collaborative plan where both parties become invested. Clients and colleagues bring background knowledge and prior experiences; capitalize on this pre-existing information. Likewise, not all clients or colleagues receive or process information in the same manner. Knowing where our client or a colleague is coming from enables the veterinary professional to directly target and tailor their message and recommendations. In this chapter, we provide communication strategies to partner with others and leverage our client's or colleagues' expertise to collectively arrive at a best plan of action. We explore two key communication skills for planning with a client or colleague: easily understood language and chunk-and-check.

SELF-ASSESSMENT QUESTIONS

1. How do I engage my clients or colleagues while planning: via a lecture or a conversation?
2. What steps do I take to tailor my recommendations to each individual client or colleague?
3. How do I present a range of options, negotiate the plan, and facilitate shared decision-making?

Introduction

Diagnostic and treatment planning conversations are the most complex of the clinical interview. What is learned during agenda-setting and information-gathering serves as the foundation on which to build the diagnostic and treatment plan (Research Spotlight 7.1). If the client's agenda is unclear, it is not possible to develop a customized plan going forward. If the history is incomplete – unstable and insecure – the structure is fragile. This could result in a lack of client commitment to the care plan, putting client satisfaction, patient health, and practice performance at risk (Sidebar 7.1). The same holds true for collegial interactions; to achieve the best outcomes, take time to understand where the team is coming from before shifting into problem-solving mode.

Developing Communication Skills for Veterinary Practice, First Edition. Jane R. Shaw and Jason B. Coe.
© 2024 John Wiley & Sons, Inc. Published 2024 by John Wiley & Sons, Inc.

Research Spotlight 7.1

Invest Time in Information-Gathering

Quantitative analysis of video-recorded veterinarian-client-patient interactions found that, on average, veterinarians spend almost 50% of their time in the clinical interview on diagnostic and treatment planning and only 10% on history-taking (Shaw et al. 2004). These findings suggest that veterinary professionals speed through information-gathering and then get bogged down during diagnostic and treatment planning. The recommendation is to instead focus on agenda-setting and information-gathering at the beginning, to meet the end goal of adherence to the care plan. This requires reallocating how time is spent and increasing information-gathering early on to streamline diagnostic and treatment planning.

Sidebar 7.1   Outcomes of Effective Diagnostic and Treatment Planning

Enhance efficiency
Increase client understanding and recall
Promote buy-in and adherence
Foster client satisfaction
Improve patient health
Boost practice performance

Front-load the appointment by fully eliciting the client's agenda and performing thorough information-gathering. Without knowing a client's or colleague's concerns, goals, expectations, and priorities, offering options or solutions is like shooting in the dark until an agreeable path forward is struck. It becomes a process of trial and error that takes considerable time. Explore information relevant to the patient, the client, and their environment to lay the groundwork for an efficient planning process. The up front investment in agenda-setting and information-gathering pays off with mutual understanding, which empowers decision-making.

Clients bring background knowledge and prior experiences with them to the appointment; capitalize on this pre-existing information. The sources are highly variable. Some clients encountered similar events with other animals or dealt with the illness in themselves, a family member, or a friend. They may research information on the internet, hear about a topic on television, or read about it in a magazine. Or they may reach out to others and discuss their concerns with friends at the dog park, their breeder, or the groomer. Other clients work in human healthcare and bring considerable medical knowledge.

Ask about client knowledge beforehand to avoid patronizing or losing clients. If the client already knows most of our spiel, we go to the next step, thereby improving appointment efficiency. If the client does not possess prior knowledge, we slow down and catch them up to where they need to be. Likewise, our colleagues join the practice with diverse circumstances, qualifications, and credentials and appreciate being hand-picked for projects and recognized for their expertise.

Not all clients and colleagues receive or process information in the same manner. Some individuals are auditory learners (i.e. learn from verbal explanations), others are visual learners (i.e. learn from reading; watching a demonstration; seeing a picture, photo, or model; or viewing the radiograph or bloodwork results), and still others are kinesthetic learners (i.e. learn from performing the procedure or participating in show-and-tell) (Leite et al. 2010). Before launching into an explanation, ascertain your client's or colleague's information preferences, to present and target messages to enhance comprehension.

Knowing where the client is coming from enables the veterinary professional to tailor information and recommendations directly to the client and patient. Then the veterinary team and client work collaboratively to leverage the veterinary knowledge (i.e. animal healthcare) and client expertise (i.e. agenda, perspective, knowledge level, and information preferences) to arrive at the best treatment option. Similarly, team leaders capitalize on their own expertise and that of their colleagues to arrive at creative solutions to difficult practice-level challenges.

In this chapter, we explore two key communication skills for planning with a client or colleague: easily understood language and chunk-and-check (Sidebar 7.2). We provide examples in three locations: in the examination room with Ms. Lin, a medical student and her cat, Felix, who is in the clinic for suspected hyperthyroidism; in a team meeting about client financial policies led by Jenna, the practice manager; and in a conversation about client financial options between Andy, a veterinary technician, and Dr. Mala, in her office.

Sidebar 7.2 Two Communication Skills for Diagnostic and Treatment Planning

Easily understood language
Chunk-and-check

Set the Scene

Client Scenario: Ms. Lin, a medical student, presents with Felix, a 10-year-old male castrated, orange, domestic short-haired cat. Felix is losing weight despite a voracious appetite and seems to be drinking and urinating more than normal. Based on history, physical examination, and bloodwork findings, Dr. Mala's diagnosis is feline hyperthyroidism.

Team Scenarios: Jenna, the practice manager, is facilitating a veterinary team meeting. The primary topic is developing a Good Samaritan fund and identifying other programs or resources for clients struggling to care for their pets and pay their veterinary bills. This item was brought to the team's attention by Andy, a veterinary technician who is passionate about providing financial assistance to clients who otherwise could not provide care for their pets. This was fueled by a conversation with Dr. Mala and Andy's desire to help Ms. Lin provide the care that Felix needs.

Stepping into Dr. Mala's and Jenna's shoes, self-reflect on:

1. How would I present the diagnostic and treatment options to Ms. Lin?
2. How would I facilitate a collaborative brainstorming meeting with my team to develop various options for client financial support?

Plan with Clients

Key Communication Skills for Diagnostic and Treatment Planning

Easily Understood Language

Definition
The use of language that is appropriate, relevant, and meaningful to the client or team member (Research Spotlight 7.2). But research suggests that we use language that clients do not understand (Medland et al. 2022). In a large marketing study, 43% of clients felt that their veterinarian did not communicate using language they understood (Bayer Healthcare 2011).

Research Spotlight 7.2

Avoid Medical Jargon

In client focus group studies, participants preferred that veterinarians communicate in lay terminology (Coe et al. 2008; Janke et al. 2021a). As these findings suggest, it is important to be mindful of using simple, clear, and succinct client-friendly language.

Technique
Pay attention to the language and word choices used by the client. Avoid medical jargon, unless appropriate, and instead use lay language or define terminology in a manner the client easily comprehends.

Examples
> *The reason Felix is hungry all the time, but still losing weight, is that he has an overactive thyroid gland, which increases his metabolism; basically, it is causing him to burn a lot of calories.* [easily understood language] ***What*** *else can I answer for you*? [open-ended inquiry]

Chunk-and-Check

Definition
An explanatory strategy in which we give information in small pieces (chunk) and then ask about client comprehension (check) before moving on. This approach provides manageable doses of information for the client to absorb while intermittently taking a pulse of the client's understanding, which guides the direction of further discussion (Silverman et al. 2013).

Technique
The purpose of chunk-and-check is to convert a lecture into a conversation, allowing time for the client to process information and pose questions. It establishes a give-and-take, back and forth dynamic and paces the discussion with the client's needs (Research Spotlights 7.3 and 7.4).

Research Spotlight 7.3

Chunk-and-Check

In-depth client interviews and focus groups found that clients wanted veterinary professionals to slow down, take time to listen, address clients' questions as they arise, and repeat information as needed (Coe et al. 2008; Stoewen et al. 2014). These communication checkpoints facilitate client comprehension and in turn improve clients' recall and adherence to recommendations, highlighting the importance of breaking down our explanations into digestible bite-size pieces.

Research Spotlight 7.4

Check for Client Understanding

Quantitative analysis of video recordings of veterinarian-client interactions found that in 34% of appointments, veterinarians did not ask for the client's understanding (Shaw et al. 2004). The finding identifies a missed opportunity to take a moment to check and assess client comprehension to reduce confusion or misunderstandings before moving on in the explanation.

1. **Chunk:** Present only one to three sentences at a time using short, easily understood phrases. Keep in mind that a digestible piece of education for a client may differ from that of the veterinary team. The client is likely to be hearing this material for the first time. If the information is bad news, unexpected, emotional, or stressful – or medically complicated or sophisticated – the client may not be able to process it at their regular speed. Therefore, even smaller and simpler bites, with prolonged pauses, may be required.

2. **Check:** Before proceeding to the next topic, check with the client: elicit questions, ask for the extent of their understanding, allow time for processing, or ascertain readiness to move on. The check could include a literal break in the conversation (e.g. maybe the client goes to lunch, takes a walk, makes a phone call, sleeps on the information overnight, or returns for a recheck visit) with a clear intention to pick it up later.

Another check technique is asking clients to restate or summarize back to us, in their own words, what they heard from the veterinary team. Exercise this skill carefully, as it could be misinterpreted if worded or presented inappropriately. With strong rapport, a nonjudgmental tone of voice, genuine curiosity, and humility, this skill is well-received by clients. Framing our request in a manner that puts the onus on us, the veterinary team, immunizes the exchange against perceived condescension.

The "check" is a powerful open-ended inquiry tool for involving clients or colleagues and gaining their perspective, as such, there are four places in this book that we refer to the check. The first was to check for remaining items during agenda-setting. The second is here to request feedback from a client or colleague after an explanation (chunk-and-check). The third is to follow-up after an internal summary to ascertain from our client's or colleague's perspective if the information is complete (Chapter 6). The last is the final check at the closing of the interaction after an end summary to assess if there are any remaining questions or comments (Chapter 8).

Examples

Felix will need to be on daily medications to control the thyroid disease. If you miss multiple doses, his symptoms will return shortly. [chunk] ***What*** *questions do you have about Felix's home care?* [check]

I've shared a lot of information with you, and I struggled with being clear. ***Would you mind*** *sharing with me* [ask permission] ***what*** *you heard?* [check – summarize back]

Attend to the Process of Diagnostic and Treatment Planning

The **how** of diagnostic and treatment planning is the communication process or the way we conduct these often challenging and complex conversations.

Foster Shared Decision-Making

Partnership leads to shared decision-making, which encourages a balance of power between veterinary professionals and clients. It is a process in which the veterinary team and client work together to make decisions. The emphasis is on the exchange of information, expression of preferences, and fostering choice between treatment options (Elwyn et al. 2012). A three-step model illustrates how to implement shared decision-making with clients (Box 7.1). There is evidence that shared decision-making is lacking in veterinary practice (Janke et al. 2021b) (Research Spotlight 7.5), and yet when both veterinarian and veterinary technician communicate with a client, it contributes to enhanced shared decision-making (Janke et al. 2022) (Research Spotlight 7.6).

Box 7.1   Put Shared Decision-Making into Practice

There are three steps to implementing shared decision-making (Elwyn et al. 2012):

1. Inform the client that there are options to consider and choices to make.

    *There are **four treatment options** to treat Felix's hyperthyroidism.* [signpost] ***Let's** review these options **together** to determine what is going to **work best for you and Felix**.* [partnership]

2. Educate the client about the advantages and disadvantages of each option, and check for the client's understanding.

    The surgical procedure is called a thyroidectomy, in which we remove the thyroid gland. We need to be cautious of nearby structures during surgery and supplement Felix with thyroid hormone afterward. [chunk] ***What** can I clarify?* [check]

3. Explore client preferences, and support deliberation to determine which option is best for the client and patient.

    ***What** are your thoughts on the options I presented?* [open-ended inquiry]
    ***What**'s important to you in making this decision?* [open-ended inquiry]
    ***How** can I best support you?* [partnership]

Research Spotlight 7.5

Share Decision-Making

A study used the observer OPTION[5] tool to measure veterinarian shared decision-making. The mean score was 23 out of 100 in 717 Canadian veterinary visits (Janke et al. 2021a). These findings indicate a wide gap between client preferences for partnership and involvement in decision-making (Janke et al. 2021b) and what is happening in veterinary practice.

Research Spotlight 7.6

Use Your Team to Enhance Shared Decision-Making

Another study using the observer OPTION[5] measure to assess veterinary professionals' contribution to shared decision-making found that decisions involving both a veterinarian and veterinary technician scored significantly higher for shared decision-making (29.5) than veterinarian-only (25.4) and veterinary technician-only decisions (22.5). With combined efforts of veterinarian and veterinary technician, there was significantly greater client education about options and integration of client preferences into the decision-making process (Janke et al. 2022). These results emphasize the important role veterinary technicians play in supporting client decision-making and the need to equip and support them for this role.

Give a Lecture vs. Have a Conversation

Diagnostic and treatment planning discussions are often unidirectional, with the veterinary professional delivering information with little to no client input. Because we possess substantial medical knowledge, it is easy to lecture; however, when we hold court, we potentially alienate and frustrate our clients. Lecturing focuses on the veterinary team's agenda of educating the client and we may lose sight of the client's concerns, perspectives, or expectations.

Our communication style influences how we deliver information (Chapter 2). As a refresher, the expert drives their agenda forward, does most of the talking, and shot-puts information that is large in mass and scale and may be difficult for the client to comprehend (Barbour 2000; Kurtz et al. 2005). To foster shared decision-making, the partner takes a collaborative approach, involves all parties, Frisbees information in small pieces targeted to the client, and elicits client feedback and responses (Barbour 2000; Kurtz et al. 2005). Clients prefer engaging in a partnership dialogue with their veterinarian (Coe et al. 2008; Janke et al. 2021a) (Research Spotlight 7.7), and there are a variety of ways to use our communication skills to invite client participation in the planning process (Box 7.2).

Research Spotlight 7.7

Be a Partner

In client focus groups, participants conveyed their desire to establish a partnership with veterinary professionals. Clients preferred that veterinarians employ two-way communication, involve them in discussing options, and work with them to make an informed decision (Coe et al. 2008; Janke et al. 2021a). Findings support the importance of engaging our client to take an active role in making decisions and caring for their pet.

Box 7.2   Techniques for Encouraging Client Participation

Use a variety of communication skills to engage clients, including a simple pause, empathy, reflective listening, asking permission, an open-ended inquiry, or a summary.

Use of silence [pause]
***What** are your **thoughts**?* [open-ended inquiry]
***Shall I** continue?* [asking permission]
*You were **not expecting** this diagnosis today.* [empathy]

(Continued)

Box 7.2 (Continued)

What questions do you have at this point? [open-ended inquiry]
I hear that Felix's health is of the utmost importance to you. [reflective listening]
*How would **you like to proceed**?* [open-ended inquiry]
*What additional information might be helpful **for you**?* [open-ended inquiry]
What concerns do you have? [open-ended inquiry]
What experience do you have with pilling cats? [open-ended inquiry]
Would it be helpful [asking permission] *to **try out the explanation on me*** [partnership] *before you explain it to your husband?* [check – summarize back]

Achieve Informed-Client Consent

One of the goals of shared decision-making is informed-client consent; to arrive there, veterinarians and clients discuss differential diagnoses, diagnostic procedures, treatment options, risks and benefits, prognosis, and costs of care (Flemming and Scott 2004, CVO 2014; AVMA 2007) (Sidebar 7.3). Veterinary professionals provide clients with enough relevant information in understandable language so they make a medically sound and practical decision for themselves and their pet (Flemming and Scott 2004). Therefore, it is critical that informed-client consent consists of a discussion, not a signature on a consent form.

Sidebar 7.3   Components of Informed-Client Consent

Patient's diagnosis
Diagnostic or treatment options
Risks and benefits
Prognosis
Costs of care
Who will perform the procedure or treatment?
Where will the procedure or treatment be performed?

Flemming and Scott (2004); CVO (2014); AVMA (2007).

During the conversation, veterinary professionals explain the risks and benefits with a forthright discourse and balance patient and client advocacy (Fettman and Rollin 2002). Our ethical obligation is to ensure that our patients do not suffer, while ensuring that all clients are treated equally and that we respect their autonomy and do not unduly influence their decisions (Yeates and Main 2010). Our role is to ensure that the client possesses the information necessary to make an informed decision.

Take a Structured, Stepwise Approach

A stepwise approach divides the decision-making process – breaking the conversation into pieces and providing information that is more easily digestible – and allows clients to reflect and process at each stage (Sidebar 7.4). We are unlikely to complete all the steps in one appointment; later steps may require follow-up appointments or phone calls. These conversations are incremental rather than linear, both during and between appointments. Clinical knowledge is developed over time, puzzle pieces fall into place, and findings become detailed and clear. Initially, there may be multiple rule-outs under consideration, and further testing may be required to reach a final definitive diagnosis.

Sidebar 7.4   Diagnostic and Treatment Planning Process

1. Present physical examination findings.
2. Outline the medical problems.
3. Give the presumptive or definitive diagnoses.
4. Present diagnostic or treatment options.
5. Discuss advantages and disadvantages.
6. Provide the prognosis.
7. Make a medical recommendation.
8. Discuss costs of care.
9. Negotiate the diagnostic or treatment plan.
10. Finalize informed-client consent.

Multiple factors may detour our stepwise process. The patient does not respond to the initial treatment, necessitating additional diagnostic tests or a different treatment approach. Or the client has financial limitations, so the diagnostic tests may be run incrementally or treatment may be based on a presumptive diagnosis. At each turn, we revisit the advantages and disadvantages. The process may even return to information-gathering to reveal key missing details and refine the diagnostic process. The ideal culmination of the conversation results in informed-client consent.

1. **Present physical examination findings.**
   Talking through the physical examination demonstrates to the client what you are doing, why it is important, and how it benefits the health of the patient. A communication gap between veterinarians and clients is a lack of client awareness of whether a physical examination was performed (AVMA 2018). Even if clients note it, they may not know what is happening during the pet's physical examination or what it means for their pet's wellbeing. This is an opportunity to advocate for our expertise and the importance of the physical examination. The *Talking Physical Exam* describes what we are doing while our hands are on the animal; we demonstrate the thoroughness of our examination while communicating the value (da Costa et al. 2022).

   > *I am gently feeling for Felix's thyroid gland in his neck. It is enlarged, which could explain his symptoms. Let me* **complete his physical exam,** [signpost] *and* **we** *can talk about what this means.* [offering partnership]

2. **Outline the medical problems.**
   The problem list is initially composed of concerns elicited during agenda-setting, information-gathering, and physical examination and then updated once diagnostic test results are available. To promote accuracy, summarize the problem list back to the client before moving forward to ensure that you are both on the same page.

   > ***Just to summarize,*** *Felix is hungry all the time, but he is losing weight; he's drinking a lot, and you have noticed larger-than-normal urine clumps in the litterbox. From my examination, his thyroid gland is enlarged.* [internal summary] ***What*** *would you like to add?* [open-ended inquiry]

3. **Give the presumptive or definitive diagnoses.**
   In presenting the potential diagnoses, think out loud with the client and share what you think are the most likely causes based on what the client is seeing, what the patient is exhibiting, and

what was found on the physical examination. The list of rule-outs is further informed by results from diagnostic testing. Be gentle but clear and direct in presenting the diagnosis. There is evidence that veterinarians may avoid discussing sensitive diagnoses (Research Spotlight 7.8).

Research Spotlight 7.8

Deliver a Direct and Clear Diagnosis

In a survey study of veterinary professionals' perceptions of discussing pet obesity with clients, 54% (55/102) avoided conducting the conversation with certain clients, depending on the veterinary professional's relationship or history with the client, especially if they sensed a lack of client readiness (Sutherland et al. 2022a). It is the veterinary professional's role to gently, directly, and honestly deliver a clear diagnosis, and it is the client's choice how to address it.

From what you shared and what I found in feeling Felix's enlarged thyroid gland and hearing his increased heart rate, it is likely that Felix has feline hyperthyroidism – an overactive thyroid gland – making him hungry, lose weight, and drink and pee more. [chunk] ***What*** *have you learned about thyroid disease in medical school?* [check]

4. **Present diagnostic or treatment options.**
   When appropriate, present a range of diagnostic or treatment options to the client and elicit their questions, thoughts, and concerns as you proceed. Offering an array ensures that you are not limiting, assuming, selecting, or biasing the choices for the client. There is evidence that veterinary professionals limit the options presented based on whether they think the client can afford them (AAHA 2003; Cron et al. 2000). This is a prerequisite for informed and shared decision-making; clients want to know their choices (Research Spotlight 7.9).

Research Spotlight 7.9

Present Multiple Treatment Options

Client focus group findings support that clients want to know the medical options available (Coe et al. 2008; Janke et al. 2021a). However, findings indicate that veterinarians provide what they perceive to be the "best" option for the client and their animal and then modify that option if necessary (Coe et al. 2008). Present clients with the menu of relevant options, and discuss them to support a shared decision-making process.

The practitioner's communication style often sways how options are presented to the client (Shaw et al. 2006). Parallel to the communication styles presented in Chapter 2, there are three different approaches to presenting diagnostic and treatment options (Box 7.3). To achieve agreement and buy-in, the key is to align closely with the client's preferences.

Box 7.3   Communication Style Impacts Presenting Options

Expert – This is the traditional approach (useful during an emergency), in which the veterinary professional takes the lead and presents their recommended option(s) based on their expertise and advocacy for the patient with an expectation that the client will comply. The options are often limited, to one: the gold standard. Challenges arise when clients feel pressured, do not agree with or adhere to the plan, or face barriers to implementation.

*I recommend treating Felix with radioactive iodine therapy. I will refer both of you to a veterinary specialist who will conduct the treatment. Let me **get** that information for you.* [signpost]

Facilitated or guided – This is a collaborative, partnership approach (useful in chronic disease or preventive care) in which the veterinary team presents all the relevant options and informs and supports the client through the decision-making process. We advocate for the needs of both the client and the patient, resulting in a mutually agreed-on plan.

If it is all right with you, [asking permission] *I am going to share with you the options available for Felix, [signpost] based on the information I gathered. **Next**, we'll explore the benefits of each [signpost] and discuss **together** which is the option for Felix and you. [partnership] At the **end**, I will **provide the cost of care** alongside each of the options. [signpost] Please ask questions for clarification along the way. **How** does that sound?* [check]

Laissez-faire – This approach lacks both leadership and guidance. The veterinary team presents all the options and leaves it up to the client to make the final decision. The assumption is that the client is equipped and wants to make the decision, which can result in a lost, overwhelmed, frustrated, or paralyzed client.

There are several considerations during this phase of the conversation. Beware of making assumptions about a client's willingness to pay and prematurely limit treatment options (AAHA 2003; Cron et al. 2000). Choose words carefully, and avoid right, best, or gold standard, as clients may feel judged if they choose an alternative treatment option. Watch nonverbal emphasis (i.e. voice tone, volume, and facial expressions), which might indicate an option preference and unduly influence the client.

*The following diagnostic tests – a complete blood count, chemistry panel, urinalysis, and thyroid profile – would allow us to confirm Felix's diagnosis and ensure that there are no other health concerns that we need to take into consideration. [chunk] **What** are your thoughts?* [check]

*Let's **review all the options** we have for treating Felix. [signpost] Then **we** can consider what would **work for you and Felix**. [offering partnership]*

5. **Discuss advantages and disadvantages.**
   It is prudent to provide the client with unbiased and transparent information about how the diagnostic test, procedure, treatment, or surgery may help or harm the patient (Research Spotlight 7.10).

Research Spotlight 7.10

Facilitate Client Informed Decision-Making

During client focus groups, participants indicated that they wanted a range of options so they could make an informed decision on behalf of their pet. They expected their veterinarian to discuss the advantages and disadvantages of each treatment option within the context of their individual animal (e.g. with respect to their animal's age, clinical signs, disease, and prognosis) as well as present the cost of each option (Coe et al. 2008; Janke et al. 2021a). Findings support the importance of taking the time to fully discuss the advantages and disadvantages of each option and tailoring the plan to the individual client and patient.

With the option of medication, some cats do very well and other's experience side effects, including vomiting, decreased energy, or not eating. A few cats are allergic to this medication and exhibit severe itching and scratching. If these signs happen, we would need to re-evaluate and likely consider another treatment. [chunk] **What** *questions do you have?* [check]

One important thing *to be aware of is that* [signpost], *for some cats, hyperthyroidism masks underlying kidney disease. What this means is that after we treat the thyroid disease and the heart rate and blood pressure return to normal, we may find, with the decreased blood flow to the kidneys, that Felix also has underlying chronic kidney disease. So, we'll regularly check his kidney function with blood tests and urine samples.* [chunk] **What** *worries you about this possibility?* [check]

6. **Provide the prognosis.**

   Discussing the prognosis is a critical conversation about what the disease and diagnosis mean for the patient's quality of life and lifespan. During this discussion, be open and honest and set realistic expectations for the caregiver regarding the possible disease trajectory and requirements for the animal's supportive care at home. Share whether the disease can be cured, only managed, or palliated, and how you will monitor the patient's response to treatment.

   Felix has a good prognosis if he receives and tolerates his daily medication, we will monitor his thyroid levels regularly, and you can watch for signs at home, such as increased energy level, appetite, drinking and peeing, or weight loss. [chunk] *To see if I've communicated clearly,* **what** *will you watch for at home?* [check – summarize back]

7. **Make a medical recommendation.**

   Clients seek the veterinary professional's medical expertise to provide guidance, so after presenting the options, it is critical to clearly present medical recommendations (Research Spotlight 7.11). There is evidence of missed opportunities for veterinary professionals to provide clear recommendations (AAHA 2003, 2009; Sutherland et al. 2022b) (Research Spotlight 7.12). This advice is based on what you learned during agenda-setting and information-gathering about the client's perspective and situation and the client's and animal's lifestyle and environment. The goal is to align the medical recommendation with the client's concerns, priorities, goals, and expectations.

Research Spotlight 7.11

Make Clear Medical Recommendations I

A quantitative study examined the association between veterinarian-client communication and client adherence to dental or surgical recommendations. The study found that client adherence was seven times greater for clients who received a clear recommendation than clients who received an ambiguous recommendation from their veterinarian (Kanji et al. 2012).

    Ambiguous recommendation: *I recommend that Felix come in to recheck his thyroid level in a little while.*

    Clear recommendation: *I recommend that Felix come in to recheck his thyroid levels in four weeks. Let me introduce you to Katya, our client coordinator, to assist you in scheduling that appointment.*

    These results emphasize the importance of making a simple, succinct, clearly stated recommendation and supporting client follow through.

Research Spotlight 7.12

Make Clear Recommendations II

In a study of 150 veterinarian-client interactions involving discussions of an obese veterinary patient, only 43% of these discussions included a weight management recommendation (Sutherland et al. 2022b). Findings of the study identify that opportunities exist to provide a clear and concrete recommendation among health care options to help clients make informed decisions.

> *Given what you shared with me, I recommend treating Felix with a daily medication. You would have a choice, as the drug comes in two forms: a pill that can be administered by mouth, or there is an ointment that you would massage into the skin topically, on the inside of his ear.* [chunk] ***What*** *are your thoughts?* [check]

8. **Discuss costs of care.**
   With each diagnostic or treatment option, provide the cost of care, which is an important component of informed-consent guidelines (Flemming and Scott 2004). Clients expect veterinary professionals to communicate costs associated with the treatment options up front (Research Spotlight 7.13), but evidence reveals that discussing cost is a challenge for many veterinary professionals (Kipperman et al. 2017) (Research Spotlight 7.14). Clients who understand the value of each option in relation to the cost are in a stronger position to make informed decisions for themselves and their animal with minimal regrets.

Research Spotlight 7.13

Discuss Cost Upfront I

During client focus groups, participants expressed a preference that the care of the patient take precedence over the veterinarian's compensation. At the same time, clients expected veterinarians to initiate cost discussions up front (Coe et al. 2007). Combining these findings, clients want financial discussions, but do not want money conversations to take priority over the care of the pet. This means it is important to present the costs of veterinary care while communicating the benefits of the care to the health and well-being of the animal.

Research Spotlight 7.14

Discuss Cost Upfront II

During a veterinarian focus group, many veterinarians shared that financial conversations are uncomfortable (Coe et al. 2007). In a 2009 follow-up study, analysis of video recordings of veterinarian-client communication revealed that financial conversations are infrequent – only

(Continued)

Research Spotlight 7.14 (Continued)

29% (58/200) of appointments included a cost discussion – and reference to a written estimate was made in only 14% (28/200) of appointments (Coe et al. 2009).

And unfortunately, not much has changed. In a 2022 study examining 917 video-recorded veterinarian-client interactions, only 24% included a cost discussion (Groves et al. 2022). These findings indicate a need to communicate the cost of veterinary care, which is an integral component of diagnostic or treatment planning and informed-client consent.

I hear that you have financial constraints and want to do all you can to make Felix better. [reflective listening] *Let's work through the options together.* [offering partnership]
I wish that cost did not come into play in caring for our pets; it is a challenging reality. [empathy] *Let me share with you* [offering partnership] *the cost of each option to be sure you have the information you need to decide.* [signpost]

9. **Negotiate the diagnostic or treatment plan.**
   Clients want what is best for their pet but may not be able to afford their preferred medical option. These discussions walk a tightrope between best-practice recommendations on one side and offering a spectrum of care on the other (Stull et al. 2018; Brown et al. 2021). The choices range from advanced, expensive treatments to less-specialized, lower-cost options.

   We often need to come up with a customized diagnostic and treatment plan that meets the client's financial constraints, perspectives, or beliefs, and living situation (Research Spotlight 7.15). During this conversation, we balance educating the client regarding care for their pet and demonstrating nonjudgmental respect for the client (Research Spotlight 7.16). Our goal is to ensure that the patient receives the care it needs, the plan fits within the client's restrictions, and the client maintains a long-standing, trusting relationship with the veterinary practice.

   The veterinary professional's role is to educate clients, facilitate the decision-making process, provide support, reduce influence, and foster informed choices. Multiple factors

---

Research Spotlight 7.15

Incorporate Client Preferences

In a focus-group study of client and veterinarian perceptions of weight-related communication, it was important to pet caregivers that veterinarians incorporate their preferences and limitations into developing realistic weight-management plans (Sutherland et al. 2022c). Clients reported frustrations with veterinarian recommendations to change physical activity that were neither appropriate nor feasible. These findings highlight the importance of eliciting the client's perspective to create a tailored plan for success.

influence client decision-making (e.g. beliefs, values, resources, and time), and a frequent one is financial constraints (Box 7.4).

Research Spotlight 7.16

Respect Client Decisions

During client focus groups, participants shared that they want veterinarians to give them a range of options, provide a medical recommendation, and respect their decision. Specifically, clients indicated they did not want to feel pressured, be told what to do, or be made to feel guilty (Coe et al. 2008; Janke et al. 2021a). Findings indicate that clients value a veterinary professional's guidance and assistance in sorting through the options that exist, without making the decision for them.

Box 7.4   Planning with Financial Limitations

Here are key steps to negotiating the diagnostic or treatment plan with a client who has financial limitations:

1. Present all available medical options, make a clear medical recommendation, and discuss the costs of care.

   *There are **several acceptable paths** we can take to ensure that Felix gets the care he needs.* [signpost] ***Let's go over** [partnership] the advantages and disadvantages of each option and the associated costs before coming to a final recommendation and decision.* [signpost]

2. Allow time for the client to reflect and process the information. Take a pause or break in the conversation or call on the client's support system. Be mindful about not taking the client's initial reaction as their final decision, as it may just be sticker shock. With some time to think it over or discuss it with other key decision makers, the client may feel differently.

   ***I hear you saying** it is expensive.* [empathy] [pause]

   ***Would you** like some time to think it over?* [asking permission]

   ***Would it be** helpful to discuss this with other members of your household?* [asking permission]

3. Check with the client to determine how they perceived the recommendation and how they would like to proceed.

   ***I appreciate** that you did not expect the expenses of the bloodwork and urinalysis today.* [empathy] ***And it sounds like** you have additional questions regarding costs.* [reflective listening] ***Tell me** your concerns.* [open-ended inquiry]

(Continued)

Box 7.4   (Continued)

It will be an investment up front to make the diagnosis and determine the medication dosage. Once Felix's thyroid levels are stable, the costs will lessen. [chunk] ***What*** *are your thoughts about proceeding?* [check]

4. Reevaluate the plan together, if the client cannot or chooses not to pursue the medical recommendation. Review the advantages and disadvantages of each diagnostic or treatment option, and explore an alternative approach that better aligns with the client's perspective or situation.

   I hear that *radioactive iodine therapy is not in your budget right now.* [reflective listening] ***Let's revisit*** *the other options to see what might* ***work for you and Felix***. [partnership]

5. Provide nonjudgmental support.

   Each of the potential options is ***worthy of our consideration*** *in treating Felix.* [empathy]

   I want you to know that there is ***no right or wrong decision***. [empathy] *Each has advantages and disadvantages.*

6. Be flexible, as there may be an out-of-the-box clinical solution; and be open to considering other potential resources.

---

10. **Finalize informed-client consent.**

    As discussed previously, informed-client consent starts with fostering a dialogue; presenting the risks and benefits of procedures while inviting client questions. Check one last time to see if there are any remaining questions or concerns. Outline clear expectations, and prepare the client for possible unintended outcome(s). If or when a medical complication arises, the client may be more understanding and trusting. This is a case where time spent up front pays off if or when an adverse event occurs. If appropriate, the final step may be a formal signature on a consent form.

Use the Value Matrix

The Value Matrix is a visual tool to present each diagnostic and treatment option, discuss the advantages and disadvantages, approximate the cost, and make a shared decision. It is a roadmap of the diagnostic and treatment options that presents the key points (Coe 2017). It also takes the form of a handout that the client brings home with them and refers to after the discussion. This unbiased, informed, efficient, and inclusive technique to present choices balances best practice recomendations with the client's perspective and financial resources. Make an important note that in using the Value Matrix, each option's value, to the client and patient, is presented **before** the financial costs. Figure 7.1 shows an example of a Value Matrix that could be used to assist a client (e.g. Ms. Lin) in making an informed decision regarding their pet's veterinary care (Box 7.5).

Warning: Keep an open mind, as this approach initially sounds time intensive. However, working through each stage answers important client questions and ultimately creates a clearer path forward, easing decision-making and alleviating confusion.

Patient and Client Benefits

Treatment Options	Outpatient Care	Minimally Invasive	Fewer Side Effects/ Complications	Less Lifelong Monitoring	Cures Hyper-thyroidism	Does Not Require Referral
Medication	✓	✓	X	X	X	✓
Dietary Therapy	✓	✓	?	X	X	✓
Surgery	X	X	X	✓	✓✓	✓/X
Radioactive Iodine Therapy	X	✓	✓	✓	✓✓	X

Key:
✓ - An advantage to the patient or client
X - A potential disadvantage to the patient or client
? - Unknown or uncertain impact

Figure 7.1 An Example Feline Hyperthyroidism Value Matrix.

Box 7.5 Steps in Building a Value Matrix

1. List all the diagnostic or treatment options **vertically** on the left-hand side of a white board to be photographed or on a sheet of paper to be handed to the client. This serves as the basis or starting point for presenting the diagnostic or treatment options.

   Here is a list of options we can consider to treat Felix's hyperthyroidism:

   a. *Medication*

   b. *Dietary therapy*

   c. *Surgical removal of the thyroid gland*

   d. *Radioactive iodine therapy*

2. List **horizontally**, across the top of the whiteboard or piece of paper, the advantages and disadvantages associated with each diagnostic or treatment option, for the patient and the client. This row often aligns with items in the client's agenda and ensures that the conversation considers the client's perspective as well as the benefits to the health and well-being of the patient.

   Let's** discuss* [offer partnership] *the potential **advantages and disadvantages** associated with each option and **address your concerns: [signpost]

   a. *Outpatient care*

   b. *Minimally invasive*

(Continued)

Box 7.5 **(Continued)**

---

   c. *Fewer side effects/complications*

   d. *No lifelong monitoring*

   e. *Cures hyperthyroidism*

   f. *Does not require referral*

3. Place a ✓ on the matrix in relation to each option that offers a respective patient or client advantage and an X where the option does not serve the patient or client. In areas of uncertainty, place a ?. This process recognizes that an advantage of one option is a disadvantage of another. In some cases, two options each benefit the patient or client, but one option's benefit is greater than the others'; therefore, you might use ✓✓ to represent the additional benefit of that option. The outcome is an illustration for the client to compare options and make a fully informed decision.

*Now, I'm going to go through **each treatment option**, I will put a ✓ for each advantage to Felix and yourself. If there's a disadvantage, I'll put an **X**; and if we are not sure, let's put a **?**. [chunk] **What** can I clarify before we proceed? [check]*

4. Use **differentiating factors** to highlight the effectiveness of the various treatment options. Look down the vertical columns to find clear distinctions between the advantages and disadvantages of each option. For example, in the feline hyperthyroidism Value Matrix in Figure 7.1, cure versus management is a critical differentiator between the options: two of the options (radioactive iodine therapy and thyroidectomy) cure feline hyperthyroidism, and the other two options (medication and prescription diet) manage the disease.

We have four options for addressing Felix's hyperthyroidism, two of which, radioactive iodine therapy and surgery, will cure Felix's hyperthyroidism. The other two options, medication and a special diet, manage his disease. [chunk] What path are you considering for Felix? [check]

5. Look across the horizontal rows for the option with the most ✓s, and the least Xs to identify the **best practice recommendation**. However, the option with the most ✓s on the Value Matrix (radioactive iodine therapy, in Felix's case) may not end up being our final recommendation.

Radioactive iodine therapy is indeed the current treatment of choice for cats with hyperthyroidism (AAFP Guidelines 2016). However, after factoring in the client's perspective, lifestyle, environment, or situation into our recommendation, we, along with our client, may arrive at a different decision. Ms. Lin, for example, expressed financial constraints, so medication may be the treatment option that fits her pocketbook and still offers a reasonable approach for controlling Felix's hyperthyroidism.

*As we can see, the most effective option for curing hyperthyroidism is radioactive iodine therapy, which targets the overactive cells in Felix's thyroid gland to stop producing too much thyroid hormone. [chunk] **What** questions do you have about that option? [check]*

6. Add in the **costs** associated with each option in the far right-hand column as a final step. Check with Ms. Lin as you go. This approach underscores the advantage (value) of each option to the patient and client before discussing the costs of care.

*Because financial matters are a consideration in decision-making, I'm going to **note the cost associated with each treatment option**. [signpost]*

7. Use the Value Matrix as a visual tool to support shared decision-making and ensure informed consent. As needed, it is used to reevaluate which option fits with the client's constraints, concerns, and beliefs while not causing undue harm to the patient.

So, it sounds like radioactive iodine therapy is not a financially feasible option. [reflective listening] *A reasonable alternative approach is to use medication to control Felix's hyperthyroidism. This is not a cure, although it will manage his hyperthyroidism, cost less up front, and in most cases keep him stable. A drawback is that it will require medication daily, and over time, costs will add up with regular monitoring of his thyroid levels for the rest of his life.* [chunk] ***What*** *are your thoughts on taking this approach?* [check]

Adapted from Coe (2017).

Attend to the Content of Diagnostic and Treatment Planning

The communication content or **what** of diagnostic and treatment planning refers to the type of information presented.

Meet as Experts

Traditionally, diagnostic and treatment planning conversations were centered on biomedical topics: problem list, differential diagnoses, diagnostic tests, and treatment options for the patient. Today, in taking a relationship-centered approach, we incorporate the client's agenda, perspective, starting knowledge, and information preferences into the planning process. Shared decision-making is a collaborative process.

The veterinary team members are experts in animal healthcare, and the client is the recognized authority in the day to day aspects of caring for their animal. So, our role is to ascertain and capitalize on the client's areas of expertise to formulate a plan that fits well for the client and the patient. This means making time to learn about the client and patient before telling them what we think is going on with their animal.

If the client remains unclear or unsure or gets stuck during decision-making, refrain from the tendency to tell them more. Instead, back up and ask questions. Doing so may uncover a physical, emotional, or ideological barrier to be overcome to jumpstart the decision-making process (Stoewen et al. 2014) (Research Spotlight 7.17).

Research Spotlight 7.17

Elicit Client Expertise

In-depth interviews with clients with dogs that were recently diagnosed with cancer revealed that clients want information to be tailored to their background, knowledge base, previous experiences, and information preferences (Stoewen et al. 2014). This means personalizing the information. Doing so was empowering for clients, and it enabled them to make treatment decisions, granted them a sense of control, and fostered their ability to cope with their dog's cancer diagnosis. When clients get stuck during decision-making (i.e. decision paralysis), take a step back to gain a greater understanding of who they are and what they need. What you learn may "unlock" the client and, at the very least, engender compassion, patience, and understanding.

The end goal is to create a mutually agreed-on plan of care that is satisfactory to the client and the veterinary team. With a partnership in place, both parties buy into the care plan and take responsibility for the decisions and associated outcomes. If or when things do not go as planned, both parties are accountable and work together toward a solution, reducing blame and finger-pointing.

Tailor the Plan to Each Client and Patient
Facilitating a true meeting of experts means tailoring the diagnostic or treatment plan to each individual client and patient. Veterinary professionals often present well-rehearsed scripts to educate clients. Customizing the diagnostic or treatment plan means modifying that spiel for each client based on what was learned during agenda-setting and information-gathering.

During the discussion, check regularly with the client and invite them to express their thoughts, ask questions, clarify key details, and express possible reservations. Listen for client cues – repeated words, phrases, questions, or concerns – that signal further explanation may be required. Based on client feedback, modify what and how you present the next piece of information. As you and the client throw the Frisbee back and forth, you fine-tune the information you are providing directly to the client's information needs (Barbour 2000; Kurtz et al. 2005).

Adapting our spiel ensures that our clients understand what we are saying. It keeps the client engaged and an active participant in the conversation. When we are effective in educating clients, we strengthen their recall and understanding and, subsequently, their investment and commitment, leading to greater client adherence to the care plan and loyalty to the practice.

Enhance Client Health Literacy
Tailoring the diagnostic and treatment plan requires accounting for an individual's health literacy; their ability to access health information.

> **Health literacy** implies the achievement of a level of knowledge, skills, and confidence to take action to improve personal and community health by changing lifestyles and living conditions. Thus, health literacy means more than being able to read pamphlets and make appointments. By improving people's access to health information, and their capacity to use it effectively, healthy literacy is critical to self-empowerment (WHO 2023).

The Program for International Assessment of Adult Competencies (PIACC) assesses literacy in adults between the ages of 16 and 65 from different countries (NCES 2020). The PIACC defines literacy as "understanding, evaluating, using, and engaging with written text to participate in society, achieve one's goals, and develop one's knowledge and potential." The tasks range from reading simple passages to complex problem-solving and are rated on six levels (below level 1 to level 5).

The first round of the PIACC assessment was conducted in 2012 and the second in 2014, and the datasets were combined into one data point for 2012/2014. The third data collection occurred in 2017, and the results are presented in Figure 7.2. The key finding is that approximately 20% of individuals are below level 1, and 30% are at level 2. This means we need to take steps to foster clients' health literacy through observations, conversations, and the use of educational tools.

There are four components to health literacy (e.g. functional, communicative, critical, and self-efficacy) (Lee et al. 2016; Shaw and Hunter 2017) (Box 7.6 and Figure 7.3). The veterinary team capitalizes on these dimensions to enhance client understanding, recall, and adherence to medical recommendations. The result is that, through improved understanding, clients are better positioned to approve diagnostic recommendations, choose treatment options, and provide the nursing care their pet needs.

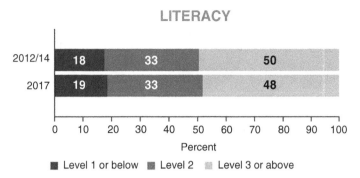

Figure 7.2 Percentage distribution of US adults aged 16–65 at selected levels of proficiency in Program for International Assessment of Adult Competencies literacy: 2012/2014 and 2017. *Source:* U.S. Department of Education, National Center for Education Statistics 2023.

Box 7.6   Components of Health Literacy

Functional literacy: Clients come into the veterinary practice with a level of comprehension of animal healthcare. The team's responsibility is to assess their level of understanding by watching for clues such as not completing paperwork, not reading (or making excuses for not reading) printed materials, or language use. Offer a translator if someone is available and equipped to do so on the veterinary team or use translation or assistive technology to support communication.

I noticed that you did not fully complete your paperwork. **Can we** *go through the questions together?* [asking permission] <*Read the questions out loud to the client.*>

Let's *see if there is a copy of this handout for you.* [partnership]

Would you prefer *if I explain using pictures or words?* [asking permission]

Communicative literacy: During the visit, the veterinary team encourages the client to engage in conversation by posing questions and asking for information to be repeated back, so at home the client communicates what is going on with the pet and presents options to other decision-makers in their household.

What *are the key points that you will share with your family?* [open-ended inquiry]

How *will you implement our plan for Felix at home?* [open-ended inquiry]

Critical literacy: The veterinary team aids clients in using information to weigh the advantages and disadvantages in considering options and making decisions.

What are the most important factors *to you in making this decision?* [open-ended inquiry]

What *do you see as the advantages and disadvantages?* [open-ended inquiry]

Self-Efficacy: With strong health literacy, clients feel empowered to take an active role and feel confident and competent (i.e. a sense of agency) in caring for their pet at home.

How *have you made important pet-care decisions in the past?* [open-ended inquiry]

You know Felix best – **how** *do you think he will respond?* [open-ended inquiry]

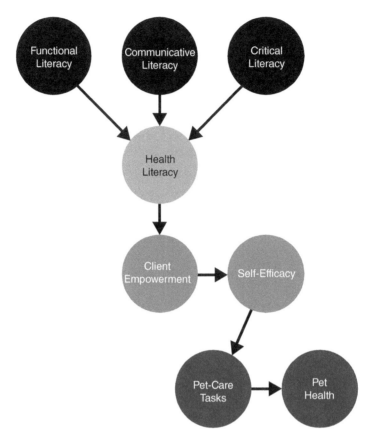

Figure 7.3 Health literacy model. *Source:* Shaw and Hunter (2017) with permission.

Avoid Medical Jargon

Enhancing health literacy entails paying close attention to language usage. In a study of discharge summaries provided to clients of pets with a recent cancer diagnosis, the written information exceeded recommended readability levels (Medland et al. 2022). There are two considerations: how a sentence is constructed (how long or short or convoluted or straightforward it is) and word choice. Almost every profession uses its own vocabulary. Just because a client does not know veterinary medical terminology does not mean they are not highly intelligent. The important thing is to communicate effectively in a way the client understands.

With a client who has a medical background, like Ms. Lin, we may be able to use precise, professional terminology such as *defecation*, *urination*, *emesis*, and *regurgitation*. Be mindful of making assumptions about a client's knowledge. Over-simplifying language for clients with medical acumen leaves them feeling offended or patronized. But using medical jargon with other clients leaves them feeling confused, alienated, or abandoned. These clients may fear coming across as ignorant or being judged if they ask for clarification or pose questions. So, strive to strike a balance between talking above or below the client's head by assessing their starting point beforehand.

Communicate Value

While it is important to present what can be done, research suggests it is even more critical to clearly outline and connect it with why it needs to be done. We need to communicate how our recommendation enhances the health and wellbeing of the patient (Research Spotlight 7.18). It is the **why** or **so what** that speaks directly to the client (Coe et al. 2007; Lue et al. 2008; AAHA 2009; Volk et al. 2011). There is evidence that "stating the why" is lacking in veterinarian-client interactions (Research Spotlight 7.19).

In the scenario of Felix, the cat with suspected hyperthyroidism, we want to run a thyroid profile on a regular basis to monitor his response to treatment. Ms. Lin will likely want to know why this regular testing is needed, how this test will help Felix, how we will use the test results to make a

---

Research Spotlight 7.18

Communicate Value

Findings from client and veterinarian focus groups suggest that veterinarians perceive "value" differently from their clients. Veterinary teams focus on the medical tangibles, such as time, specialized equipment, and professional services provided – what they can do for the animal (Coe et al. 2007). In contrast, the **why** is what is most important to clients – how will this recommendation benefit the health and wellbeing of their pet (Coe et al. 2007; Lue et al. 2008; AAHA 2009; Volk et al. 2011)?

Research Spotlight 7.19

State the Why

In studies examining veterinarian-client interactions containing a cost conversation, veterinarians discussed the cost of services in relation to the benefit to the patient's health and well-being in only 17% (10/58) (Coe et al. 2009) and 14% (31/215) (Groves et al. 2022) of the interactions. Similarly, in a study of 150 obesity-related veterinarian-client discussions, in only 28% (42/150) of the conversations did the veterinarian provide the client with a reason for pursuing weight management (Sutherland et al. 2022b). These findings validate when making recommendations to include both what you can do and, most importantly, how and why it will help the pet.

---

diagnosis, how it will inform our treatment recommendations, and how it will help Felix feel better or stay healthy for the long term.

> *I appreciate that the initial diagnostic tests and the regular monitoring **add up**.* [empathy] *By closely monitoring, we can keep an eye on Felix's thyroid levels. If we become concerned, we can adjust his medications to reduce the potential impact on Felix's heart and kidneys. Regular monitoring will help us keep him healthier in the long run.* [chunk] ***How*** *might that work for you?* [check]

Manage Client Uncertainty

Uncertainty is core to a client's experience of an animal's illness. Two methods were identified to reduce client uncertainty: meeting clients' informational and/or relational needs (Stoewen et al. 2019). Our "go-to" when a client is struggling to understand is often to provide more information. However, what the client may really want is emotional support. When clients are uncertain, ask yourself if they need education or listening, empathy, and partnership (Research Spotlight 7.20).

Research Spotlight 7.20

Support Uncertain Clients

During in-depth interviews of clients with dogs with cancer, uncertainty was identified as a dominant client psychological experience (Stoewen et al. 2019). Traditionally, the veterinary team focused on treating the animal's disease. The results of this study highlight the importance of the veterinarian's role in supporting how the client copes with the animal's illness.

Delivering informational support involves giving hospital orientations and tours, providing information aligned with client preferences, forewarning about difficult news, and conducting open and honest conversations about expectations and prognosis (Stoewen et al. 2019). The focus is empowering the client through equipping them with information.

Providing relational support means building a trusting relationship with the client. Minimize client distress by offering timely service when booking appointments, scheduling tests and procedures, communicating results, and returning phone calls. Expand client care by encouraging peer and family support through interactions in the waiting room, social communities (among family, friends, or neighbors), and/or via formal internet groups (Stoewen et al. 2019). The emphasis is on empowering clients through making connections with the veterinary team and extending client-support resources.

Commonly Asked Questions Related to Diagnostic and Treatment Planning

What Happens If the Client Cannot Afford to Provide Care for the Patient?

These are challenging conversations for both clients and the veterinary team. Client economic limitations affect the veterinary team's ability to provide desired care for patients and contribute to burnout (Kipperman et al. 2017). Clients who are unwilling to pay (8.3%) and low-income clients (6.9%) are common practice-based stressors for veterinary professionals (Van de Griek et al. 2018). Moral stress results when veterinary professionals grapple with wanting to do what is best for our patients, but are prevented from doing so. It is ethically challenging when we cannot provide the life-saving medical care we were trained to administer (Kahler 2015).

Sometimes difficulties arise, and a compromise cannot be reached. This requires out-of-the-box thinking with the client and veterinary team to research community and professional resources. Options to explore include relinquishment, a Good Samaritan fund, using a credit card for healthcare expenses, referral to a subsidized-care clinic, the Humane Society or Animal Protection League, rescue or breed organizations, grateful client donations, or veterinary financial relief funds. In some cases, euthanasia may be the most humane choice to end animal suffering. Although this is a devastating outcome for the client and veterinary team, the informed and collaborative decision-making process may ease the veterinary team's and client's guilt, regrets, and resentment.

How Do I Simultaneously Present Myself as Both an Animal Healthcare Expert and a Partner?

Some veterinary professionals perceive partnership as wishy-washy or unstructured and prefer more control with shot-putting. Many believe that if the client takes the lead – grabs the Frisbee and runs with it – the veterinary professional will be left behind. This misperception is a source of discomfort and reluctance to partner with clients. With a partnership, we maintain our role as the animal healthcare expert and client educator. Clients bring their own expertise and share their perspective, knowledge, background, and preferences; the key is collaboration.

What does collaborative diagnostic or treatment planning look like? At each step – presenting treatment options, discussing advantages and disadvantages, making a medical recommendation, and going over costs – the veterinary team advises the client and invites them to ask questions, contribute their thoughts, make their own informed decisions, and maintain client autonomy. The big difference is that we engage the client in a dialogue, elicit and respect the client's perspective, and integrate the client's concerns into our recommendations. The result is a meeting of experts; the veterinary team in animal healthcare and the client in all aspects of their and the pet's lives.

Who on the Veterinary Team Discusses the Cost of a Diagnostic or Treatment Plan?

Using the Value Matrix to present treatment options requires a certain level of medical knowledge. In most instances, the veterinarian is in the strongest position to facilitate the cost conversation and outline the advantages and disadvantages for the patient to the client. This said, there are common preventive-care conversations (e.g. vaccination, deworming, flea, tick, and heartworm prevention, elective surgeries, dentistry, behavior, nutrition, and obesity management) that other members of the veterinary team can be trained to handle. The bottom line is that the person who presents the diagnostic and treatment options needs to be equipped to discuss the cost of veterinary care with clients and, most importantly, the benefits to the health and wellbeing of the pet.

How Do I Find Time for a Complete Diagnostic or Treatment Planning Discussion?

Gathering the client's full agenda and history prepares all parties for diagnostic or treatment planning and sets up a more efficient process. Knowing the client's agenda and perspective enables us to tailor our treatment recommendations to them, accelerating the decision-making process and securing client buy-in. Obtain a complete picture of the situation – including patient, client, and environment data – and identify potential barriers to the plan.

Assessing the client's knowledge, previous experiences, and information preferences guarantees that our message is targeted to the individual on initial delivery, thus reducing the need for clarification. These steps prevent wasting time educating clients on information they already know or focusing on an option that will not work for them. Chunk-and-check is the critical skill we use to gauge the client's response and identify reservations or misunderstandings on the spot to promptly address them.

How Do I Present the Treatment Options before I Have a Confirmed Diagnosis?

Depending on the clinical scenario, it is overwhelming for the client to process so much information at one time. Or the list of differential diagnoses may be vast and difficult to narrow down, and predicting treatments may be too convoluted. One way to handle this situation is to ask permission from the client.

> *Although we do not yet have a confirmed diagnosis,* **would you like me to** *go over potential treatment options with you today or wait until we have results?* [asking permission]

Subject to the client's response, you may be able to stage the conversation. Inform the client of the potential options and then, when more information is available, provide further updates as the diagnosis is confirmed. One reason to discuss treatment options up front is that the client may not be interested in taking next steps. It is important to identify this possibility early on and not put the animal through unnecessary testing or the client through unwarranted expenses.

Routine Client Scenario

Set the Scene: Dr. Mala presented the feline hyperthyroidism Value Matrix to Ms. Lin, outlining the possible treatment options. Based on the information gathered from Ms. Lin and Dr. Mala's medical expertise, Dr. Mala made a medical recommendation of radioactive iodine therapy for Felix's hyperthyroidism.

> **DR. MALA:** *So, we covered several treatment options, the advantages and disadvantages of each, their costs, and I've made my recommendation.* [chunk] ***What*** *are your thoughts?* [check]
>
> **MS. LIN:** *What would happen if we do not treat Felix's hyperthyroidism?*
>
> **DR. MALA:** *I am fearful that Felix will continue to deteriorate and lose body weight due to increased metabolism, and I'm worried about the long-term impact on Felix's heart function.* [pause]
>
> **MS. LIN:** *How do the treatments work?*
>
> **DR. MALA:** *That's an excellent question. With the radioactive iodine therapy, eliminating the overactive thyroid cells, and thyroidectomy, the surgery to remove the thyroid gland, we could cure Felix. With the medication and the specialized diet, we can often manage the thyroid disease with a good quality of life.* [chunk] ***What*** *route are you thinking you would you like to take?* [open-ended inquiry]
>
> **MS. LIN:** *With medication, how long does Felix need to be on it?*
>
> **DR. MALA:** *He'll need to be on the medication, and we will need to regularly monitor his thyroid levels, for the rest of his life.* [chunk] ***What*** *other questions do you have?* [check]
>
> **MS. LIN:** *What if Felix has a reaction to the medication?*
>
> **DR. MALA:** *Felix could have a reaction, such as vomiting, diarrhea, or a skin rash. If that happens, we will care for him* [partnership] *and likely need to change our treatment approach.* [chunk] ***How*** *does that sound to you?* [check]

Challenging Client Scenario

Set the scene: Ms. Lin decided to put Felix on thyroid medication and came in regularly for rechecks to monitor thyroid levels, and Felix responded well. Then, one year later, Ms. Lin presents to Dr. Mala with Felix for decreased appetite and energy level, inappropriate urination, and polyuria and polydipsia.

> **MS. LIN:** *I thought you said the medication would treat this.*
>
> **DR. MALA:** *I hear your* ***frustration****.* [empathy] ***Unfortunately****,* [warning shot] *I am* ***concerned*** *that this may be a new problem like kidney disease or diabetes because Felix has responded well to the treatment for a year now.* [chunk] ***What*** *are your thoughts?* [check]
>
> **MS. LIN:** *[Sigh] I know that Felix is not doing well, and I know you'll want to do more tests. I just do not think I can afford it!*

DR. MALA: *I can only imagine how **worried** you are about Felix, and I appreciate that cost is a **concern**.* [empathy] ***Before proceeding*** [signpost] *with any tests or treatment, **we** will review our options and the costs **together**.* [partnership]

MS. LIN: *As much as I love him, I do not think I can do it. All the veterinary visits in the past year set me back with overdue bills. And what will this mean for Felix if he has another disease?*

DR. MALA: *I appreciate that this is a very **stressful** time.* [empathy] *If it's a urinary tract infection, it is something that we can address at a controlled cost. If it is kidney disease or diabetes, it will be far more complicated.* [chunk] ***What** other concerns do you have?* [check]

MS. LIN: *There is only so much that both of us can take.*

DR. MALA: *You've **worked hard** caring for Felix in the past year.* [empathy] *In coming in today, **what** are your goals for you and Felix?* [open-ended inquiry]

Talk through Technology – Self-Informed Clients

Self-informed clients are individuals who conduct research on their pet's health concerns by consulting friends and family, breeders and groomers, and other medical professionals and using the vast volume of information available on the internet. Their efforts indicate their preference for partnership and to play an active role in their pet's care. Clients seek information to educate themselves, quell fears, calm nerves, or take some control over an overwhelming experience (Sidebar 7.5). Many clients feel helpless when their pet is ill, and we address their concerns by equipping them with clear, credible information.

Sidebar 7.5   Clients Seek Information Online To . . .

Understand the pet's illness
Acquire baseline knowledge to advocate for personal and pet needs
Learn best through reading
Organize thoughts, feelings, and questions
Process a pet's diagnosis
Validate their concerns
Confirm the veterinarian's information
Answer questions not addressed in the appointment
Increase involvement in their pet's care
Seek social support from people with similar experiences
Gain control of an overwhelming scenario
Save money on a veterinary visit
Provide direct care for their pet

Adapted from Hunter and Shaw (2014).

Self-informed clients are often perceived as a challenge, hindrance, or obstacle to patient care (Coe et al. 2008; Janke et al. 2021a). However, we harness the client's desire for information and empower them to take an active role in their pet's health. Engaged clients are more likely to adhere to recommendations and provide high-quality care for their pets. When communicating with informed clients, listen sincerely and explore what they read and learned (Box 7.7). Consider client resourcefulness an asset, as there are ample opportunities to involve, educate, and energize self-informed clients to become an integral part of their pet's treatment plan.

Box 7.7   Empowering Self-Informed Clients

Use communication skills to empower, validate, and support self-informed clients:

1. Thank the client.

   Thank you for being so invested in Felix's medical care and seeking information about his thyroid disease.

2. Invite the client to share what they learned.

   What *did you learn that you'd like to share with me?* [open-ended inquiry]
   What *concerned you most from your reading?* [open-ended inquiry]
   What *questions came up during your research?* [open-ended inquiry]

3. Listen to and explore the client's perspective.

   What *is it about Felix's treatment that is most important to you?* [open-ended inquiry]

4. Ascertain the source.

   I'm always curious about what resources are available on the internet. ***Would you mind*** *sharing where you read this?* [asking permission]

5. Admit personal limits, if appropriate.

   Thank you for sharing. I have not read about that and ***would like to learn more before*** *including this therapy in our treatment plan.* [signpost] *I'd like to do some reading and consult a colleague.* [signpost] ***Can I*** *get back to you by the end of the week?* [asking permission]

6. Ask permission.

   Would you be willing *to hear my concerns about this information?* [asking permission]
   Would you be open to *reading a journal article or handout that I have found to be a reliable reference?* [asking permission]

7. Offer partnership.

   Working together, I'd like to *get you the information you desire and answer all your questions about caring for Felix.* [partnership]

8. Share tools to empower the client.

   Here's a list of websites that I've reviewed and that provide reliable information. [chunk] ***What*** *other guidance can I provide?* [check]
   There are also a couple of online support groups that other clients have found helpful. [chunk] ***How*** *does that sound to you?* [check]

9. Provide the medical diagnosis using the appropriate terminology while defining what it means in client-friendly language so that the client can research their pet's diagnosis.

   The search term you can use in your research is "feline hyperthyroidism." [chunk] ***What*** *additional information would be helpful to you?* [check]

Adapted from Hunter and Shaw (2014).

Client Education Tools

More educational tools are at our fingertips to enhance client understanding and recall than ever before. Clients prefer information to be presented in varied ways (Research Spotlight 7.21). Choosing the best tools for the client's learning style is likely to improve client comprehension, buy-in, and recall as well as adherence to treatment recommendations. As a starting point, ascertain the client's information preferences.

Research Spotlight 7.21

Using Multiple Formats

In client focus groups, participants expected information to be presented in various formats, including written discharge instructions, handouts, pamphlets, or client education packets to meet their needs (Coe et al. 2008; Janke et al. 2021b). Ask clients their preferences for additional information to support their understating, and bring those resources into the examination room with you.

In addition to handouts, treatment plans, discharge statements, and brochures, today there are white boards, screens, and computers in examination rooms. These high-fidelity tools enable showing educational videos, photographs, drawings, and three-dimensional models as well as blood test results and diagnostic images to promote visualization and client understanding. Virtual technology with enhanced imagery allows clients to tour their animal's body to see the broken bone, the tumor in the body cavity, or the disease changes in the kidney or liver. Despite the bells and whistles, a simple picture or drawing is still often highly effective in getting the message across.

Plan with the Team

Attend to the Process of Team Planning

The **how** of team planning is the communication process or the way we conduct these challenging and complex conversations. Colleagues prefer a conversational approach to planning versus lecturing. Since they are experts, they want to bring their thoughts, ideas, and experiences to the table during these sessions. In doing so, we capitalize on the collective wisdom of the veterinary team to come up with more creative and innovative solutions to problems.

The two communication skills introduced earlier in the chapter (i.e. easily understood language and chunk-and-check) support collaborative conversations during team planning. Given various educational backgrounds and levels of veterinary experience, be mindful of using medical jargon and abbreviations that may be unfamiliar. As team members bring assorted skillsets, assess colleagues' starting points and what they bring to the discussion (e.g. *What are your thoughts, experiences, or ideas?*). Get a sense of how each team member learns by eliciting their information preferences to optimize their professional development (i.e. reading, writing, auditory, verbal, or kinesthetic), and provide the resources and tools they need to grow. Actively engage colleagues in conversations by not only providing information but also inviting their contributions, assessing their understanding, and seeking out their opinions (chunk-and-check).

When facing complicated problems, take a stepwise structured approach to break a complex process into manageable pieces. Doing so ensures a thoughtful and purposeful approach; think through one step at a time, and do not skip key decision points or decision-makers. Start by developing a list of problems or challenges, identify contributing factors and potential solutions, outline the gains and losses, consider associated costs and budget impacts, negotiate a final plan, and move forward with it.

The Value Matrix is an equally useful tool to structure the planning process for team-based decisions. List the potential solutions in a vertical column and the advantages and disadvantages in a horizontal row across the top. Next, discuss the advantages and disadvantages, placing a ✓ for the most gain and X for the most loss. Then, as a team, identify what differentiates the various options.

Finally, add a column that incorporates resources required, including financial costs, personnel expertise, equipment, or time. This approach invites collaboration, tracks the decision-making process, and results in pictorial evidence of the most effective outcome (i.e. the most ✓s). As with our clients, what appears at first to be the perfect option might not be feasible or realistic for the practice or team, so alternative approaches may need to be explored.

Attend to the Content of Team Planning

The communication content or **what** of team planning refers to the type of information presented. Many of the same concepts of planning discussions with our clients apply to conversations with our colleagues. Colleagues appreciate a partnership approach – they are invited to contribute and share their ideas and expertise to foster a meeting of experts.

The diverse knowledge, skills, background, and experiences of veterinary team members require developing a customized, tailored plan for onboarding, training, and mentoring for professional development. This entails identifying everyone's areas of strength and opportunities for growth; their existing skillset, education, and areas of certification or specialization; and their learning style, and then crafting a mutual plan that enables them to succeed. Our colleagues' backgrounds differ greatly, and each brings unique skills and perspectives to the table, so meet them where they are for optimal performance.

In the day to day hustle and bustle of practice, it is easy to become task-focused – what needs to get done and how we will get it done. We may miss out on sharing the **why** – the importance, justification, or rationale – for investing time, resources, and energy in the project. It is the why that motivates our colleagues and gives a greater sense of purpose. It directly connects to how we are making a difference in the lives of our colleagues, clients, and patients. Make time to identify, share, and state the collective why.

Just like our clients, when the veterinary team faces uncertainty, they may need more information or emotional support. Our role as practice leaders is to conduct a needs assessment and fill in the data or relational gaps. Providing answers is our natural tendency, but what our colleagues may really need is a listening ear, a caring heart, or warmth and compassion.

Routine Team Scenario

Set the Scene: Jenna, the practice manager, initiates the weekly team meeting, and the main topic for discussion is the client financial policy.

> **JENNA:**   *Our **primary agenda item** today is revisiting the financial policy*. [agenda setting] ***What** else would you like to add to today's staff meeting agenda?* [open-ended inquiry] *Andy, since you raised this topic, **why don't you start** [signpost] by **sharing your thoughts***. [open-ended inquiry]
>
> **ANDY:**   *I'm interested in developing a Good Samaritan fund so we can help our clients with financial limitations*. [chunk] *I'm curious:* (he turns and addresses the rest of the veterinary team) ***what** do you all think about this option?* [check]

A colleague: *How will we determine which clients receive this type of assistance?* [open-ended inquiry]

ANDY: *That's an important consideration – there are a lot of details we need to hammer out together.* [chunk] *How do you think we could approach this?* [check]

JENNA: *This is an important idea. How do you think we could get practice leadership involved?* [open-ended inquiry]

ANDY: *I'm wondering whether we create a program draft and then present it to leadership to review and provide feedback. I'd be glad to do the research.* [chunk] *What do you think about that approach?* [check]

Challenging Team Scenario

Set the Scene: Dr. Mala presented the diagnostic test options and potential treatments including their associated costs to Ms. Lin to determine the cause of Felix's most recent deteriorating health.

MS. LIN: *I may have to put Felix down so he does not suffer.*

DR. MALA: *Would it be helpful to brainstorm ideas on how to support you, care for Felix, and to finance his veterinary care?* [asking permission] *If so, let me pull some materials together* [signpost] *for us to review.* [partnership]

While Dr. Mala is in her office assembling a folder of financial alternatives, Andy, the veterinary technician, says to her, *I cannot believe Ms. Lin is not going to treat Felix. She should not own a cat.*

DR. MALA: *This is a difficult situation for all of us.* [empathy] *Can I share with you all that Ms. Lin and Felix have been through in the last year?* [asking permission]

ANDY: *Can we ask Ms. Lin to relinquish Felix?* [asking permission] *I know we can take care of him here at the hospital.* [chunk] *What do you think about that?* [check]

DR. MALA: *That is a kind and compassionate offer.* [empathy] *What ideas do you have for covering the time and cost of Felix's care?* [open-ended inquiry]

ANDY: *The only option is for someone to adopt Felix directly and take financial responsibility for his care.* [chunk] *How would that work?* [check]

DR. MALA: *Would you be willing to adopt him and pay for his medications or find someone who will?* [asking permission]

ANDY: *I'm in no better position than Ms. Lin; I have kids who are relying on me. We must save Felix, though!*

DR. MALA: *I hear the concern in your voice.* [empathy] *We both want to be able to save Felix.* [partnership] *What other options might we consider?* [open-ended inquiry] *Let's put our heads together for Felix!* [partnership]

Put the Planning Skills into Practice

Do-It-Yourself Exercises

Exercise 7.1   Rewording Medical Jargon

The following medical terms are related to Felix's hyperthyroidism case scenario. For each term, write a short description using client-friendly, easily understood language. See examples of suggested language at the end of the chapter.

1. Thyroid gland

2. Hyperthyroidism

3. Polyuria and polydipsia

4. Lethargy

5. Inappetence

6. Inappropriate urination

Exercise 7.2 Back Pocket, Check Questions to Ask Clients

It is easy to default to the check questions *Does that make sense?* and *Do you have any questions?* Not only are these closed questions, but the phrasing biases a yes and no responses, respectively. Instead, use open-ended inquiry to elicit the client's input, not just a head nod. To expand your repertoire, brainstorm five open-ended check questions on to a piece of paper and post the list somewhere you will see it often, as a reminder. Examples of open-ended check questions are given at the end of the chapter.

Exercise 7.3 Skill Spot – Insert a Check

One of our biggest challenges is providing too much information; too large a chunk for a client to absorb and understand. In the following explanation, identify where you would insert one or more check questions and write out the open-ended check questions you would pose. See the suggested placements and check questions at the end of the chapter.

Hyperthyroidism results from an over-producing thyroid gland in the front of the neck. It increases the cat's metabolism, which is why Felix is restless, hungry all the time, and losing weight. To diagnose hyperthyroidism, we need to collect a blood sample from Felix and submit it to the laboratory to meas-ure his thyroid levels. If his thyroid levels are high, that confirms the diagnosis of hyperthyroidism. We have four options to treat hyperthyroidism, two of which cure the disease – radioactive iodine therapy and surgery – and two that manage the disease – medication and a special diet.

Exercise 7.4 Self-Assessment

Depending on your practice role, choose the most appropriate interaction to reflect on with a client or a colleague. Give yourself a quick litmus test after a recent appointment or colleague one on one, small group, or team meeting using the following reflective questions. Look at an entire con-versation, or hone in on one skill at a time. Partner with a colleague and ask them to observe and provide feedback using the following questions as a framework.

1. How did you present the information – via lecture (shotput) or conversation (Frisbee)?

2. How did you tailor the conversation to your client's or colleague's perspective, starting knowl-edge, or information preferences?

3. How did you avoid using or translate jargon?

4. How did you present your recommendation – how could you make it more clear or less ambivalent?

Exercise 7.5   Next Steps for Success

1. Based on what you learned from the self-assessment exercise, identify opportunities for growth by prioritizing one of the two communication skills – easily understood language or chunk-and-check – to focus on for a solid week. Note the results, and then add the other skill the following week to expand your repertoire.

2. Identify a coaching partner in the practice. Inform them of your communication goal, invite them to observe your interactions, and request balanced, descriptive, and detailed feedback.

3. Be gentle and kind to yourself, as initially, trying a new communication skill will be awkward and take effort until it becomes automatic and authentic.

4. Repeat the cycle of honing in on one communication skill, practicing, requesting feedback from a colleague, and conducting your own self-assessment until you achieve competence.

Engage-the-Entire-Team Exercises

Exercise 7.6   Role-play (Adapted from Hunter and Shaw 2012)

To try on the two communication skills (easily understood language and chunk-and-check), recruit two colleagues to role-play. Often, roleplaying feels forced, so you may lose focus and not take the task to heart. To remedy this, be realistic by using an empty exam room to role-play a client interaction. Conduct this exercise in three rounds, so everyone plays the role of the veterinary team member, client, and observer.

Veterinary team member role: Bring along visual aids, diagnostic images, blood results, handouts, diagrams, or discharge statements that you might use to enhance your interaction. Commit to using the communication tools as you would during an actual interaction with a client.

Client role: When taking on the role of client, respond appropriately, taking care to let the team member know whether their explanation becomes unwieldy. Look out for big chunks of information and opportunities to pause and ask questions. Do your best to provide in-the-moment feedback in the client role (i.e. offer verbal and nonverbal cues). Remember, the goal is to support your peer's development rather than being a tough client.

Observer role: As the observer, carefully watch the interaction; "Eye spy" for how your colleague uses the two communication skills and makes notes of key words, questions, or phrases offered by the client; Use the earlier self-assessment questions to serve as a notecard or checklist for this exercise.

Round 1

Veterinary team member role: Provide an explanation of feline hyperthyroidism (or a topic of your choice) employing the two communication skills.

Client role: Put yourself in the client's shoes and respond naturally and appropriately to the information provided.

Observer role: Observe how your colleague uses the two communication skills and make notes of key words, questions, or phrases offered by the client in response.

Feedback

Veterinary team member role: Share your self-reflection about what worked well and what you might try in the future.

Client role: Provide feedback on what it was like to receive the information. What worked well? What suggestion do you have to further enhance the delivery and foster dialogue?

Observer role: Give specific, detailed, descriptive feedback based on your observations and notations of the two communication skills.

Round 2

Now switch roles.

Veterinary team member role: Present diagnostic options for feline hyperthyroidism (or the topic of your choosing) using the two communication skills.

Client role: As described in round 1.

Observer role: As described in round 1.

Feedback

As described in round 1.

Round 3

Switch roles again.

Veterinary team member role: Present treatment options for feline hyperthyroidism (or the topic of your choosing) using the two communication skills.

Client role: As described in round 1.

Observer role: As described in round 1.

Feedback

As described in round 1.

Summary and debriefing

1. As a group, reflect on the exercise:
   a. What were the key lessons learned?
   b. What enhanced client understanding?
   c. What barriers prevented client understanding?
2. Assess your use of the two communication skills:
   a. How did these tools work for each of you?
   b. What went well? What might you like to try next time?
3. Develop a learning plan, and set goals for applying this experience to your day to day interactions with clients:
   a. What communication skill are you working on?
   b. How will you put it into practice?
   c. How will you assess your progress or receive feedback on your performance?

Exercise 7.7   Practice Using the Value Matrix with a Clinical Case Scenario (Adapted from Coe 2017).

1. Access key resources:

    a.   Box 7.5, "Steps in Building a Value Matrix"

    b.   Flipchart or whiteboards and appropriate markers

2. Divide the team into small groups of four or five individuals.

3. Identify common case scenarios at your practice: e.g. dental prophylaxis, overweight cat, pruritic dog, urinary tract infection, or vomiting dog (such as foreign body ingestion).

4. Choose one case scenario that the large group would like to work on.

5. Ask each small group to create a Value Matrix for the clinical scenario. The groups will work on developing a Value Matrix for the same clinical presentation.

6. Invite each group to present their Value Matrix to the team and make a clear recommendation to the client.

7. Debrief the exercise with the entire team:

    a.   What worked well? What was challenging?

    b.   How were the Value Matrices alike? Where did they diverge?

    c.   What were the medical recommendations? How did they differ?

    d.   How can the entire team work together to align differences identified between groups?

    e.   How did the Value Matrix process differ from your current approach?

    f.   How can you strengthen the consistency of your value message (benefit to the client and patient)?

8. Close with a commitment from each veterinary team member.

    a.   As a result of this exercise, what will you try moving forward?

Exercise 7.8   Practice Using the Value Matrix with a Practice- or Team-Based Scenario

1. Access key resources:

    a.   Box 7.5, "Steps in Building a Value Matrix"

    b.   Flipchart or whiteboards and appropriate markers

2. Divide the team into small groups of four or five individuals.

3. Choose a current practice- or team-based challenge, project, or relevant decision (e.g. changing the schedule, hiring a new employee, purchasing a piece of equipment, renovating clinical space, or developing a new procedure or protocol).

4. Choose one scenario that the large group would like to work on.

5. Ask each small group to create a Value Matrix for this scenario. The groups will work on developing a Value Matrix for the same practice- or team-based challenge.

6. Invite each group to present their Value Matrix to the team and make a recommendation for moving forward.

7. Debrief the exercise with the entire team:
   a. What worked well? What was challenging?
   b. How were the Value Matrices alike? Where did they diverge?
   c. What were the recommendations? How did they differ?
   d. How can the entire team work together to align differences identified between groups?
   e. What is the final decision for the team?
   f. How did the Value Matrix process differ from your current approach?
   g. How can you strengthen the consistency of your value message (benefit to the veterinary team, practice, clients, or patients)?
8. Close with a commitment from each veterinary team member.
   a. As a result of this exercise, what will you try moving forward?

Take It Away

1. **Use easily understood language,** and match your vocabulary to that of your client or colleague. Define medical terminology in client- or colleague-friendly language, and supply simple and succinct descriptions to enhance recall and understanding.
2. Foster an interactive and conversational approach, **provide information in small chunks,** and **check for understanding**.
   a. Pausing between chunks allows clients or colleagues to digest the information before moving on to the next topic.
   b. Checking for understanding or summarizing back encourages clients or colleagues to raise questions and concerns, identifying what information needs to be added, repeated, or clarified.

Answer Key

Exercise 7.1   Rewording Medical Jargon

1. Thyroid gland – Gland in the front of the neck that controls energy use in the body
2. Hyperthyroidism – An overproducing thyroid gland, which is a gland in the front of the neck, which is causing increased energy use in the body. This explains why you are seeing increased appetite with weight loss.
3. Polyuria and polydipsia – Drinking a lot and peeing a lot
4. Lethargy – Decreased energy
5. Inappetence – Decreased appetite
6. Inappropriate urination – Peeing outside the litterbox

Exercise 7.2   Back Pocket, Check Questions to Ask Clients

1. What questions do you have?
2. What can I clarify for you?

3. What additional information would you like?

4. What concerns do you have at this stage?

5. What are your thoughts on how we might proceed?

Exercise 7.3   Skill Spot – Insert a Check

1. *Hyperthyroidism results from an over-producing thyroid gland in the front of the neck. It increases the cat's metabolism, which is why Felix is restless, hungry all the time, and losing weight.* [chunk] ***What*** *questions do you have about hyperthyroidism?* [check]

2. *To diagnose hyperthyroidism, we need to collect a blood sample from Felix and submit it to the laboratory to measure his thyroid levels. If his thyroid levels are high, that confirms the diagnosis of hyperthyroidism.* [chunk] ***How*** *do you feel about proceeding with that test?* [check]

3. *We have four options to treat hyperthyroidism, two of which cure the disease – radioactive iodine therapy and surgery – and two that manage the disease – medication and a special diet.* [chunk] ***What*** *option would you like to start with discussing more?* [check]

References

American Animal Hospital Association (2003). *The Path to High Quality Care: Practical Tips for Improving Compliance*. Lakewood, CO: American Animal Hospital Association.

American Animal Hospital Association (2009). *Compliance: Taking quality care to the next level: A report of the 2009 AAHA Compliance Follow-Up Study*. Lakewood, CO: American Animal Hospital Association.

American Association of Feline Practitioners (2016). 2016 AAFP guidelines for the management of feline hyperthyroidism. *J. Feline Med. Surg.* 18: 400–416. https://doi.org/10.1177/1098612X16643252.

American Veterinary Medical Association (2007). AVMA adopts policy on informed consent. https://www.avma.org/News/JAVMANews/Pages/070515e.aspx (accessed 20 March 2023).

American Veterinary Medical Association (2018). Study shows communication gaps between veterinarians and clients. https://www.avma.org/blog/study-shows-communication-gaps-between-veterinarians-and-clients (accessed 1 December 2023).

Barbour, A. (2000). *Making contact or making sense: functional and dysfunctional ways of relating.* In: *Humanities Institute Lecture 1999–2000 Series*. Colorodo: University of Denver.

Bayer HealthCare LLC (2011). Bayer Veterinary Care Usage Study.

Brown, C.R., Garrett, L.D., Gilles, W.K. et al. (2021). Spectrum of care: more than treatment options. *J. Am. Vet. Med. Assoc.* 259 (7): 712–717. https://doi.org/10.2460/javma.259.7.712.

Coe, J.B., Adams, C.L., and Bonnett, B.N. (2007). A focus group study of veterinarians' and pet owners' perceptions of the monetary aspects of veterinary care. *J. Am. Vet. Med. Assoc.* 231 (10): 1510–1517. https://doi.org/10.2460/javma.231.10.1510.

Coe, J.B., Adams, C.L., and Bonnett, B.N. (2008). A focus group study of veterinarians' and pet owners' perceptions of veterinarian-client communication in companion animal practice. *J. Am. Vet. Med. Assoc.* 233 (7): 1072–1080. https://doi.org/10.2460/javma.233.7.1072.

Coe, J.B., Adams, C.L., and Bonnett, B.N. (2009). Prevalence and nature of cost discussions during clinical appointments in companion animal practice. *J. Am. Vet. Med. Assoc.* 234 (11): 1418–1424. https://doi.org/10.2460/javma.234.11.1418.

Coe, J.B. (2017). *Lunch and learn guide: Conveying value*. Coe Consulting.

College of Veterinarians of Ontario (2014). Guide to the professional practice standard: Informed client consent. www.cvo.org (accessed 20 March 2023).

Cron, W.L., Slocum, J.V., Goodnight, G.B., and Volk, J.O. (2000). Executive summary of the Brakke management and behavior study. *J. Am. Vet. Med. Assoc.* 217 (3): 332–338. https://doi.org/10.2460/javma.2000.217.332.

da Costa, J.C., Coe, J.B., Blois, S.L., and Stone, E.A. (2022). Twenty-five components of a baseline, best-practice companion animal physical exam established by a panel of experts. *J. Am. Vet. Med. Assoc.* 260 (8): 923–930. https://doi.org/10.2460/javma.21.10.0468.

Elwyn, G., Frosch, D., Thomson, R. et al. (2012). Shared decision making: a model for clinical practice. *J. Gen. Intern. Med.* 27: 1361–1367. https://doi.org/10.1007/s11606-012-2077-6.

Fettman, M.J. and Rollin, B.E. (2002). Modern elements of informed consent for general veterinary practitioners. *J. Am. Vet. Med. Assoc.* 221 (10): 1386–1393. https://doi.org/10.2460/javma.2002.221.1386.

Flemming, D.D. and Scott, J.E. (2004). The informed consent doctrine: what veterinarians should tell their clients. *J. Am. Vet. Med. Assoc.* 224 (9): 1436–1439. https://doi.org/10.2460/javma.2004.224.1436.

Groves, C., Janke, N., Stroyev, A. et al. (2022). Discussion of cost continues to be uncommon in companion animal veterinary practice. *J. Am. Vet. Med. Assoc.* 260: 1844–1852. https://doi.org/10.2460/javma.22.06.0268.

Hunter, L. and Shaw, J.R. (2012). 4 Courses at a 5-Star Restaurant: Explanation and Planning: Part 1. May/June: 44–49.

Hunter, L. and Shaw, J.R. (2014). The self-informed client. *Veterinary Team Brief.* September: 22–23.

Janke, N., Coe, J.B., Sutherland, K.A.K. et al. (2021a). Evaluating shared decision-making between companion animal veterinarians and their clients using the observer OPTION5 instrument. *Vet. Rec.* 189 (8): e788. https://doi.org/10.1002/vetr.778.

Janke, N., Coe, J.B., Bernardo, T.M. et al. (2021b). Pet owners' and veterinarians' perceptions of information exchange and clinical decision-making in companion animal practice. *PLoS One.* 16 (2): e0245632. https://doi.org/10.1371/journal.pone.0245632.

Janke, N., Shaw, J.R., and Coe, J.B. (2022). Veterinary technicians contribute to shared decision-making during companion animal veterinary appointments. *J. Vet. Med. Assoc.* 260 (15): 1993–1200. https://doi.org/10.2460/javma.22.08.0380.

Kahler, S.C. (2015). Moral stress the top trigger in veterinarians' compassion fatigue: veterinary social worker suggests redefining veterinarians' ethical responsibility. *J. Am. Vet. Med. Assoc.* 246 (1): 16–18.

Kanji, N., Coe, J.B., Adams, C.L., and Shaw, J.R. (2012). Effect of veterinarian-client-patient interactions on client adherence to dentistry and surgical recommendations in companion-animal practice. *J. Am. Vet. Med. Assoc.* 240 (4): 427–436. https://doi.org/10.2460/javma.240.4.427.

Kipperman, B.S., Kass, P.H., and Rishniw, M. (2017). Factors that influence small-animal veterinarians' opinions and actions regarding cost of care and effects of economic limitations on patient care and outcomes and professional career satisfaction and burnout. *J. Am. Vet. Med. Assoc.* 250 (7): 785–794. https://doi.org/10.2460/javma.250.7.785.

Kurtz, S., Silverman, J., and Draper, J. (2005). *Teaching and Learning Communication Skills in Medicine.* London: CRC Press.

Lee, Y.J., Shin, S.J., Wang, R.H. et al. (2016). Pathways of empowerment perceptions, health literacy, self-efficacy, and self-care behaviors in glycemic control in patients with type 2 diabetes mellitus. *Pat. Ed. Couns.* 99 (2): 287–294. https://doi.org/10.1016/j.pec.2015.08.021.

Leite, W.L., Svinicki, M., and Shi, Y. (2010). Attempted validation of the scores of the VARK: Learning styles inventory with multitrait multimethod confirmatory factor analysis models. *Educat. Psychologic. Measur.* 70 (2): 323–339. https://doi.org/10.1177/0013164409344507.

Lue, T.W., Pantenburg, D.P., and Crawford, P.M. (2008). Impact of the owner-pet and client-veterinarian bond on the care that pets received. *J. Am. Vet. Med. Assoc.* 232 (4): 531–540. https://doi.org/10.2460/javma.232.4.531.

Medland, J.E., Marks, S.L., and Intile, J.L. (2022). Discharge summaries provided to owners of pets newly diagnosed with cancer exceed recommended readability levels. *J. Am. Vet. Med. Assoc.* 260 (6): 657–661. https://doi.org/10.2460/javma.21.09.0410.

Shaw, J.R. and Hunter, L. (2017). Promote mutual understanding, improve client compliance. *Veterinary Team Brief.* May: 37–40.

Shaw, J.R., Adams, C.L., Bonnett, B.N. et al. (2004). Use of the Roter interaction analysis system to analyze veterinarian-client-patient communication in companion animal practice. *J. Am. Vet. Med. Assoc.* 225 (2): 222–229. https://doi.org/10.2460/javma.2004.225.222.

Shaw, J.R., Bonnett, B.N., Adams, C.L., and Roter, D.L. (2006). Veterinarian-client-patient communication patterns used during clinical appointments in companion animal practice. *J. Am. Vet. Med. Assoc.* 228 (5): 714–721. https://doi.org/10.2460/javma.228.5.714.

Silverman, J., Kurtz, S., and Draper, J. (2013). *Skills for Communicating with Patients.* London: CRC Press.

Stoewen, D.L., Coe, J.B., MacMartin, C. et al. (2014). Qualitative study of the communication expectations of clients accessing oncology care at a tertiary referral center for dogs with life-limiting cancer. *J. Am. Vet. Med. Assoc.* 245 (7): 785–795. https://doi.org/10.2460/javma.245.7.785.

Stoewen, D.L., Coe, J.B., MacMartin, C. et al. (2019). Identification of illness uncertainty in veterinary oncology: Implications for service. *Front. Vet. Sci.* 6: 147. https://doi.org/10.3389/fvets.2019.00147.

Stull, J.W., Shelby, J.A., Bonnett, B.N. et al. (2018). Barriers and next steps to providing a spectrum of effective health care to companion animals. *J. Am. Vet. Med. Assoc.* 253 (11): 1386–1389. https://doi.org/10.2460/javma.253.11.1386.

Sutherland, K.A., Coe, J.B., and O'Sullivan, T.L. (2022a). Exploring veterinary professionals' perceptions of pet weight-related communication in companion animal veterinary practice. *Vet. Rec.* 192 (4): e1973. https://doi.org/10.1002/vetr.1973.

Sutherland, K.A., Coe, J.B., Janke, N. et al. (2022b). Veterinary professionals' weight-related communication when discussing an overweight or obese pet with a client. *J. Am. Vet. Med. Assoc.* 260 (6): 1076–1085. https://doi.org/10.2460/javma.22.01.0043.

Sutherland, K.A., Coe, J.B., Janke, N. et al. (2022c). Pet owners and companion animal veterinarians' perceptions of weight-related veterinarian-client communication. *J. Am. Vet. Med. Assoc.* 260: 1697–1703. https://doi.org/10.2460/javma.22.03.0101.

U.S. Department of Education, National Center for Education Statistics, Program for the International Assessment of Adult Competencies (PIAAC), U.S. PIAAC 2017, U.S. PIAAC 2012/2014. https://nces.ed.gov/fastfacts/display.asp?id=69#:~:text=The%20percentage%20of%20U.S.%20adults,in%202017%20was%2048%20percent (accessed 1 December 2023).

Van de Griek, O.H., Clark, M.A., Witte, T.K. et al. (2018). Development of a taxonomy of practice-related stressors experience by veterinarians in the United States. *J. Am. Vet. Med. Assoc.* 252 (2): 227–233. https://doi.org/10.2460/javma.252.2.227.

Volk, J.O., Felsted, K.E., Thomas, J.G., and Siren, C.W. (2011). Executive summary of the Bayer veterinary usage study. *J. Am. Vet. Med. Assoc.* 238 (10): 1275–1282. https://doi.org/10.2460/javma.238.10.1275.

World Health Organization. (2023) Improving health literacy. World Health Organization. https://www.who.int/activities/improving-health-literacy (accessed 1 December 2023).

Yeates, J.W. and Main, D.C. (2010). The ethics of influencing clients. *J. Am. Vet. Med. Assoc.* 237 (3): 263–267. https://doi.org/10.2460/javma.237.3.263.

8

Closing-the-Interaction

Abstract

Closing-the-interaction leaves a lasting impression on clients as they depart the practice, or on colleagues as they head out from a meeting. What happens during the closing is a testament to the orchestration of all the previous steps in the clinical interview: opening-the-interaction, information-gathering, attending to relationships, attending to tasks, and diagnostic and treatment planning. The goal is to come to an efficient, succinct, mutual agreement. Our approach to the closing influences whether clients or colleagues go through with the plan, follow up, and return. In this chapter, we explore communication tools for setting up our clients or colleagues for the next critical step, the successful implementation of the plan. We explore three communication skills for closing-the-interaction with a client or colleague: end summary, contracts for next steps, and final check.

SELF-ASSESSMENT QUESTIONS

1. How do I formally close an interaction with a client or colleague?
2. How prepared are clients or colleagues to take next steps at the end of a discussion?
3. How often during the closing do new client or colleague concerns arise?

Introduction

Like opening-the-interaction, on the face of it, the closing seems deceptively simple. The closing leaves a lasting impression on clients as they depart the practice or colleagues as they head out from a meeting. We hope to conclude the appointment with time for expressions of gratitude; however, endings often feel rushed, regardless of diligent preparation.

What happens during the closing is truly a test of the orchestration of all the previous steps in the clinical interview – opening-the-interaction, information-gathering, attending to relationships, attending to tasks, and diagnostic and treatment planning. Based on the questions clients are asking, we may suddenly realize that they did not understand or absorb the information we provided. We may find our hand on the doorknob when the client drops an "oh, by the way" bomb. Most of the problems that arise during the closing stem from missed opportunities – cues or issues the client raised earlier in the appointment that the veterinary professional overlooked or neglected to pursue (Research Spotlight 8.1).

Research Spotlight 8.1

Oh, By the Way

We presented these findings in Chapter 3, and they warrant revisiting in the closing, as this is when "oh, by the way" moments occur. A study looking at veterinarians' solicitation of client concerns during the opening of an appointment found that the odds of a new concern arising at the end of the appointment were four times greater when the veterinarian did not fully elicit the client's concerns during the opening (Dysart et al. 2011). Not getting the full agenda upfront increases the potential of the client (or colleague) raising important information, including hidden concerns, later in the visit, leading to potentially longer appointment or meeting times. So, based on these findings, it is important that we take a few critical minutes at the beginning of the visit to fully elicit our client's or colleague's agenda.

The late-arising agenda item is a painful lesson learned from not fully eliciting the client's agenda at the beginning of the appointment (Dysart et al. 2011). The reverberations are felt by all team members – client coordinators handling frustrated clients in the lobby, veterinary technicians struggling to maintain the appointment schedule, and veterinarians pressured to get back on track. Slowing down during opening-the-interaction and obtaining the client's full agenda makes for smooth sailing at the closing.

Client or colleague uncertainty, confusion, or frustration at the end of the interview or meeting is a sign that we missed a key ingredient during the interaction, such as not identifying an important client's or colleague's perspective, offering time to ask questions, or seeking agreement with the plan (Sidebar 8.1). In posing a final check at the closing, we hope the client, or our colleague brings up nothing new. If something does come up, acknowledge and address it, as this is the intention of the final check before the client or colleague departs dissatisfied.

Sidebar 8.1   Start from the Beginning

Employ these communication skills early in the interview to successfully close the interaction:

Agenda-setting
Reflective listening
Open-ended inquiry
Pause
Internal summary
Empathy
Partnership
Asking Permission
Signpost
Chunk-and-check

When under pressure, we often default to lecturing to make up for lost time, and we abandon the partnership created with carefully crafted communication. A similar phenomenon occurs when we run out of time at the end of a team meeting; we speed up to get through the agenda. We may dig a deeper hole when we were hoping to end on a high note.

While closing-the-interaction, we set up our client or colleague for the next critical step; the successful implementation of the plan. The closing determines whether they go through with the plan, follow up, and return. One of the goals of the closing is to come to an efficient, succinct, and mutual agreement (Sidebar 8.2).

Sidebar 8.2   Clinical Outcomes of Closing-the-Interaction

Enhance client recall and understanding
Improve adherence
Increase client satisfaction
Grow client retention
Foster patient health
Boost practice performance

In this chapter, we explore three communication skills for closing-the-interaction with a client or colleague: end summary, contracts for next steps, and final check (Sidebar 8.3). We provide examples in two locations: in the examination room with Dr. Barbara Dalton, who is working with the Ellis family and their dog, Bruno; and with Shaquita, the practice manager, who is conducting annual performance reviews with Shaina, a client service supervisor, and Rafael, a veterinary technician.

Sidebar 8.3   Three Key Communication Skills for Closing-the-Interaction

End summary
Contracts for next steps
Final check

Set the Scene

Client Scenario: Mr. and Mrs. Ellis rescued Bruno, a two-year-old male castrated, black Labrador retriever, from the shoulder of a rural freeway a year ago. Bruno was emaciated, tick-ridden, and bald due to mange, and the Ellis family rehabilitated him back to good health. Today, Bruno is here to see Dr. Barbara Dalton for his annual wellness visit. The formerly skinny dog morphed into an obese Labrador (Hunter and Shaw 2012).

Team Scenario: Shaquita, the practice manager for a five-doctor practice, scheduled an afternoon of back-to-back annual performance reviews. Mid-afternoon, she meets with Shaina, a client service supervisor, who is exceeding expectations and seeking opportunities for promotion. The last review is with Rafael, one of the veterinary technicians, who struggles with project management responsibilities and does not know how to resolve the issue.

Stepping into Dr. Dalton's and Shaquita's shoes, self-reflect on:

1. In closing-the-interaction, how would you ensure that the Ellis family has no remaining questions or concerns regarding Bruno's agreed-on weight management plan?
2. In closing the performance review with Shaina or Rafael, how would you highlight the key points from the review?

Closing Client Interactions

Key Communication Skills for Closing-the-Interaction

End Summary

Definition

Reflecting two or more items at the closing that draws together the most salient points for the client and highlights the take-home information. A checkpoint to ensure that we are not missing key information and that everyone is ready to end the visit. Using an end summary effectively ties together data, observations, and findings and confirms key take-away messages for the client.

Technique

An end summary pulls together two or more pieces of data, and it involves two steps. The first is presenting an explicit synopsis, followed by a check, which allows the client to respond to, add to, correct, or clarify; this is achieved through a long pause or posing an open-ended inquiry. Sidebar 8.4 provides examples of phrasing to begin a summary statement that was also provided in Chapter 6 in discussing internal summary.

Sidebar 8.4   Summary Stems

To recap . . .
To summarize . . .
To pull it all together . . .
To make sure I have it all . . .
Let me see if I am correct . . .
Let me see if I got this right . . .
What I heard is . . .
What you are saying is . . .

Example

> **Moving forward,** *you agreed to put Bruno on a special diet to be measured out twice a day, replace treats with green beans, and take him on a 20-minute walk, once or twice a day.* [end summary] **How** *are you feeling about all this?* [open-ended inquiry]

Contracts for Next Steps

Definition

A process for outlining the roles and responsibilities of the veterinary professional and the client moving forward. Summary and contracting statements are often confused. Summary is what was discussed (in the past), and contracting is what is going to happen next (projects into the future). Often, veterinary professionals move quickly into contracting, forgetting to take a minute to summarize the key points of the visit first.

Technique

This is an explicit statement defining what the veterinary professional will do and the client's tasks. Include contingency plans: let the client know what to do if things do not go as planned, how to prepare for unexpected outcomes, and how to seek help.

Example

> **Would it work for you** to bring Bruno in once a month for a weigh-in to track his progress? [asking permission] *We will make changes as needed until he reaches his ideal body weight.* [contracts for next steps]

Final Check

Definition

An open-ended inquiry at the close of the interaction to ensure that all concerns are fully addressed and understood. It is the last confirmation that you and the client are on the same page before moving forward.

Technique

Pose an open-ended inquiry to see if there are any remaining questions, concerns, or issues for discussion. It is tempting to use a closed-ended inquiry at this stage (e.g. **Do** *you have any questions?* **Is** *there anything else?* or **Are** *there any other concerns?*). Beware as the phrasing of these closed questions biases a no response. An open-ended inquiry is more likely to coax out information, as it invites even the most reticent clients to share any items not yet covered.

Examples

> **What** *questions do you have?*
> **How** *are you feeling about our plan?*
> **What** *do you think about going forward from here?*
> **What** *would you like to add?*
> **How** *does that all sound?*

Commonly Asked Questions Related to Closing-the-Interaction

Do I Need to Summarize Yet Again at the Closing? It seems Redundant.

It does seem redundant, and that is the exact function of summary: to reflect what was said to check for accuracy, completeness, and final additions before contracting for next steps. The end summary ensures that the puzzle pieces are in the correct place and allows for clarification before moving forward. It is an efficient and protective checkpoint to catch any missing information before going ahead with diagnostic, therapeutic, or preventive care procedures.

How Do I Handle an "Oh, By the Way" Moment When It Arises?

A closing conundrum for veterinary professionals is the "oh, by the way" moment. It is the veterinary professional's role to balance the conflicting needs of the practice, veterinary team, client, and patient in addressing this challenge. This is not an easy task; there is no one good answer, and most are fraught with complications:

1. Ignore the client's concerns is a weak option. We risk jeopardizing the patient's health and client rapport, satisfaction, and trust.
2. Start information-gathering all over again, and let time management and the appointment schedule go. This route impacts the current client's experience, the next client's satisfaction, and the stress level of the veterinary team.
3. Request a drop-off of the pet to allow time for a more in-depth examination of the pet or for a procedure. Delegate to the treatment team and continue to see appointments. This is a possible

compromise, yet there is a risk of missing key information from the client, increasing the potential for misdiagnosis or mistreatment.

4. Slate a follow-up phone conversation when appointments are done for the day. Doing so makes for a very long day and less-than-ideal timing for clinical reasoning. This approach may address what the client wanted to share or learn but requires follow-up for the pet.

5. Schedule another visit or a recheck visit. This is another possible compromise; however, it may not be medically advisable, feasible, or appropriate for the patient or client to wait to be seen.

6. Solicit the client's full agenda at the start of the appointment is ideal to pick up on the client concerns and cues, and elicit the client's perspective throughout the appointment to avoid an "oh, by the way" moment at the end.

Routine Client Scenario

Set the Scene: At the four-month recheck appointment, Bruno has not lost weight. During information-gathering, Dr. Dalton reviews Bruno's exercise routine and diet history and identifies that daily walks are challenging and that Bruno is getting a measured amount of diet dog food but still receiving a lot of high-calorie dog biscuits. Dr. Dalton works with the Ellis family throughout the appointment to revise their approach to Bruno's weight-loss plan and is now in the process of closing the recheck appointment.

> **DR. DALTON:**   *So, you're doing a great job measuring out the new diet kibble. To accommodate your schedule, we are going to change daily walks to at least three times per week. The green beans were not working for you, so we're going to replace your current treats with low-calorie biscuits.* [end summary] ***How*** *do you feel about our new plan?* [open-ended inquiry]
>
> *Bruno currently weighs 94 pounds. We are going to* ***work together*** [partnership] *to bring him down to 90 pounds in four weeks.* ***We'll see*** [partnership] *how it's going in a month, at his next weigh-in, and we can adjust from there.* [contracts for next steps]
>
> ***What*** *more can I offer to help you be successful?* [final check]
>
> **MR. ELLIS:**   *We'll get this under control, Dr. Dalton, for Bruno's sake. Thank you.*

Challenging Client Scenario

Set the Scene: At the five-month weigh-in, Bruno lost four pounds; however, at the six-month weigh-in, he gained six pounds. During information-gathering, Dr. Dalton learns that the grandkids are staying for the summer and love to give Bruno treats. Dr. Dalton continues to work with the Ellis family to develop a revised plan that incorporates their new situation.

> **DR. DALTON:**   *In summary*, *it's been an eventful summer for you and Bruno. It is great to spend time with your grandkids and involve them in Bruno's weight-loss plan. I like engaging your grandkids in playing fetch with Bruno and giving him ice cubes instead of dog biscuits.* [end summary and pause]
>
> *Let the contest begin! If Bruno loses weight, we will come up with a prize for your grandkids at the end of the summer. I'll see you and your grandkids in one month for Bruno's weigh-in.* [contracts for next steps]
>
> ***What*** *other questions do you have for me?* [final check]
>
> **MR. ELLIS:**   *Dr. Dalton, do you think that giving Bruno a little piece of toast at breakfast or a few potato chips from time to time really makes a difference?*

Talk Through Technology – Emails and Texts Following an Interaction

Written communication is ripe for misunderstandings. It is easy to read too much or not enough into messages because we rely solely on the words. We provide tips below for reducing miscommunication:

1. **Watch the tone**. Unfortunately, we interpret the tone of a written message without the non-verbal cues that guide us in face-to-face conversations. It is easy to come off as abrupt. So, choose words and punctuation wisely, and read the message out loud before sending it. If in doubt, ask someone to review and interpret the message ahead of time.

2. **Provide a subject line.** With so many emails to wade through, provide a clear subject line to allow for easy search and detection. Keep it short, provide the pet's name, and clearly label the content (i.e. appointment reminder, bloodwork results, discharge instructions, or vaccinations due).

3. **Keep it short**. State the purpose of the email or text up front, and at the end, clearly identify next steps. Make the message easy to read, with clear, succinct sentences; use numbering or bullets, and allow for white space. If you are writing paragraphs, take it as a sign to pick up the phone or schedule an in-person appointment for a conversation.

4. **Proofread.** With the best intentions, we dash off a response, move too quickly, and send messages with typos, misspellings, and grammatical errors. These errors reflect poorly on us and the practice's reputation, so take a minute to read and review the text or email before pressing send. Be mindful of using medical abbreviations that clients may not understand. Make sure messages are the best reflection of what the practice represents.

5. **Think twice**. Before hitting "Reply All" or forwarding a message, pause to consider the consequences. Who will see this message? Who is the message intended for? Scroll down to thoroughly review what information is included before sharing it with others.

6. **Let it breathe.** At times, we receive email or text messages that trigger us emotionally. Perhaps we perceive someone as frustrated with us; we may be tired, impatient, or overwhelmed; or we misinterpret their underlying intention due to limited nonverbal communication. Let these messages "breathe" in the inbox and return to them in a few hours or the next day. After reflection or rereading the message, it may "sound" different. Then respond objectively, reducing the chances of escalating or misconstruing a situation.

7. **Leave no trace.** Written communication is not confidential, lasts forever, and serves as a record in court. This emphasizes the importance of the previous points of choosing technology and words wisely, proofreading, and responding rather than reacting. Text and email messages are important communication documentation to be incorporated into the medical record.

8. **Be agile**. When one mode of communication is not working, be flexible and turn to another that may be more effective. Growing frustrated when responding to the third or fourth round of texts or emails with a client or colleague may be a signal that it is time to schedule a recheck appointment or pick up the phone.

Closing Team Interactions

It is equally important to make time to properly close our colleague interactions. In informal chats we check to see if there is anything else on our colleague's mind before moving on. In formal meetings, we summarize key points, identify action items, and check for other's thoughts before concluding.

An effective closing reflects the the efficacy of the proceeding communication steps - from opening-the-meeting, agenda-setting, information-gathering to action planning. If these steps flow well, it's unlikely for a new item to arise at the closing. If we miss a step, it may require revisiting a topic and the price tag is losing meeting efficiency.

The three closing communication skills – end summary, contracts for next steps, and final check – are equally effective in tying up a one-on-one, small group, or a practice team meeting. They ensure that everyone is on the same page, clarify action items, and finalize roles and responsibilities moving forward. They also invite remaining comments and identify loose ends missed during the discussion. Everyone leaves the meeting knowing what to expect and what to do next to promote follow-through (Sidebar 8.5).

Sidebar 8.5   Practice Outcomes of Closing-the-Interaction

Enhance recall and understanding
Improve buy-in
Increase team coordination
Foster team satisfaction
Boosts practice performance

Routine Team Scenario

Set the scene: Shaquita, the practice manager, scheduled annual performance review meetings one after the other this afternoon. Her third meeting is with Shaina, a client service supervisor, who is exceeding expectations in all areas and seeking opportunities for promotion. Shaquita finished delivering balanced feedback to prepare Shaina for promotion.

> SHAQUITA: *As I shared, you are performing exceedingly well in all your job responsibilities. The area for growth is supervision and management. I mentioned the potential for a promotion in the coming year, and you sounded interested in pursuing that opportunity.* [end summary]
> *To prepare you for the promotion, I'm going to investigate some management courses, and you are going to seek out a conflict management course.* [contracts for next steps]
> *What else would you like to discuss today?* [final check]
> SHAINA: *That's all! It sounds like we have a solid plan moving forward, and I really appreciate it.*

Challenging Team Scenario

Set the Scene: Shaquita's last performance review of the day is with Rafael, a veterinary technician, with a history of not completing projects in a timely manner. It is the end of the day, and both are growing tired. Shaquita delivers balanced feedback on Rafael's performance, and they brainstorm how to address Rafael's challenge of completing projects.

> SHAQUITA: *To wrap up, the items that we discussed **working on together** [partnership] in the coming year are identifying a continuing education program to grow your interest in offering hospice care for our patients and improving the efficiency of your project management by outlining tasks and setting deadlines at the beginning.* [end summary] *What other topics did we miss?* [open-ended inquiry]

*As a starting place, **let's** [partnership] create a list of your current projects with status updates, priority designations, and realistic deadlines. Then **we can** [partnership] review things together on a weekly basis.* [contracts for next steps] **How** *does that sound?* [open-ended inquiry]

What *else do you need from me to prepare for our next meeting in a week?* [final check]

RAFAEL: *I don't know where to start. Can you repeat what you want me to do again?*

Put the Closing Skills into Practice

Do-It-Yourself Exercises

Exercise 8.1   Skill Spot – The Closing
Label the closing communication skill – end summary, contracts for next steps, or final check – for each of the following examples. The answer key is posted at the end of this chapter.

1. *What other concerns do you have today?*

2. *You shared that meeting deadlines has always been a challenge for you, and we brainstormed working together to outline steps and set priorities for your projects.*

3. *How else can I help you today?*

4. *We will see you in a month for another weigh-in. In the meantime, you are going to continue to measure out the diet food, stop feeding table scraps, give only green beans for treats, and take Bruno for daily morning walks.*

5. *It sounds like you are doing a great job measuring the diet dog food and giving green beans for treats. Bruno's weight gain seems to come down to getting more treats from the grandkids, which we now have a plan to address.*

Exercise 8.2   Self-Assessment
As the key communication skills for closing-the-interaction fall into place, do a quick litmus test after a recent client or colleague interaction using the following questions:

1. How satisfactory was the closing for you, and why?

2. How clearly was the plan summarized?

3. How did the final plan outline responsibilities for both parties moving forward?

4. What "oh, by the way" issues arose at the end of the interaction, and why?

Exercise 8.3   Next Steps for Success
Based on lessons from the self-assessment, identify opportunities for growth, and prioritize the order in which to work on the closing communication skills (end summary, contracts for next steps, and final check).

1. Choose one of the three communication skills and focus on it for a solid week. Note the results, and then add another to your closing repertoire the following week.

2. Identify a coaching partner in the practice. Share your communication goals, invite them to observe your interaction with a client or colleague, and request balanced, descriptive, and detailed feedback on your closing of the interaction.

3. Be gentle and kind to yourself, as initially, trying new communication skills is awkward and takes effort until they become automatic.

4. Repeat the cycle of focusing on one communication skill, practicing, and requesting feedback from a colleague until you feel you succeed in regularly using each of the three skills for closing-the-interaction.

Take It Away

1. **Summarize** frequently and often throughout the clinical interview, including a formal **end summary** at the closing to ensure that everyone leaves the interaction on the same page. This is an important review of information to obtain agreement and commitment to the plan.

2. **Contracts for next steps** to outline what will happen next, so both parties are aware of their roles and responsibilities in implementing the plan.

3. **Final check** is the last chance to confirm that your client's or colleague's concerns are addressed, elicit any remaining questions, and offer an important checkpoint before formally closing-the-interaction.

Answer Key

Exercise 8.1   Skill Spot – The Closing

1. *What other concerns do you have today?* [final check]

2. *You shared that meeting deadlines has always been a challenge for you, and we brainstormed working together to outline steps and set priorities for your projects.* [end summary]

3. *How else can I help you today?* [final check]

4. *We will see you in a month for another weigh-in. In the meantime, you are going to continue to measure out the diet food, stop feeding table scraps, give only green beans for treats, and take Bruno for daily morning walks.* [contracts for next steps]

5. *It sounds like you are doing a great job measuring the diet dog food and giving green beans for treats. Bruno's weight gain seems to come down to getting more treats from the grandkids, which we now have a plan to address.* [end summary]

References

Dysart, L.M.A., Coe, J.B., and Adams, C.L. (2011). Analysis of solicitation of client concerns in companion animal practice. *J. Am. Vet. Med. Ass.* 238 (12): 1609–1615. https://doi.org/10.2460/javma.238.12.1609.

Hunter, L. and Shaw, J.R. (2012). On-time departure: Closing the consultation. *Veterinary Team Brief.* September/October: 30–34.

9

Communication Coaching

Abstract

Coaching is a purposeful set of skills for developing, empowering, and cultivating others; the coach supports colleagues in improving performance. It is employed to develop clinical, technical, or professional skills, and anyone within the veterinary practice, regardless of role, can be trained to serve as an effective coach. A key process is that the colleague, rather than the coach, sets the direction, objectives, and expectations for the work, and the coach serves as a facilitator. In this chapter, we present a communication coaching process and identify opportunities for observation, feedback, self-reflection, and ongoing communication skill practice. The components of a coaching session include a briefing (objective-setting) and an observed client or colleague interaction (performance), followed by debriefing (self-reflection and feedback). Opportunities for communication coaching abound in the clinic setting, using role-play, video review, peer-observation during appointments, or work shadowing. Applying lessons from this book, we discuss using the communication skills introduced in the previous chapters for the communication coaching of colleagues.

SELF-ASSESSMENT QUESTIONS

1. Which best describes my natural coaching style: to be curious and ask questions, or to provide answers and give direction?
2. How do I like being coached by my colleagues: being guided in finding the answer myself, or being told what needs to be done?
3. How well does my communication style align with the partner style used for coaching?

Introduction

A paradigm shift is occurring in veterinary practice leadership. The traditional commanding approach is evolving into a more collaborative one. Many employees, no longer content with being passive, prefer to take an active role on the team. Individuals in the workplace today desire to be valued as team members and recognized for their contributions (Moore et al. 2014).

Concerns for professional wellbeing in the veterinary profession highlight the importance of creating high performing and functioning veterinary teams that work efficiently together in a

Developing Communication Skills for Veterinary Practice, First Edition. Jane R. Shaw and Jason B. Coe.
© 2024 John Wiley & Sons, Inc. Published 2024 by John Wiley & Sons, Inc.

compassionate and supportive practice culture (Moore et al. 2014; Pizzolon et al. 2019). To shift to a teamwork approach, we need to turn the top-down hierarchical structure in veterinary practice on its head. In its place, we invite team members to sit at the table and take part in brainstorming, problem-solving, and decision-making (Kinnison et al. 2014) (Sidebar 9.1).

Sidebar 9.1 Outcomes of Effective Coaching

Promote professional development
Foster staff engagement
Improve job satisfaction
Prevent burnout
Strengthen staff retention
Increase practice performance

This requires an equal shift in our colleagues' mindsets. If we take a growth perspective – seeing failure as educational and assessment as an investment in our professional development – then we will all be more receptive to feedback. On the other hand, with a fixed mindset, we see our traits as static and immobile, and feedback is perceived as threatening and met with defensiveness. Individuals in a growth state of mind embrace coaching and in a fixed state of mind may resist coaching.

Coaching is a purposeful mentoring or teaching style to develop, empower, and cultivate others; the coach supports colleagues in improving performance. Coaching is employed to develop clinical, technical, or professional skills, and anyone within the veterinary practice, regardless of role, can be trained to serve as an effective coach. A key process is that the colleague, rather than the coach, sets the direction, objectives, and expectations for the work, and the coach serves as a facilitator.

In communication coaching, specifically, we apply our communication skills, use a coaching process, and create opportunities for observation, feedback, self-reflection, and ongoing practice (Sidebar 9.2). The components of a coaching session include a briefing (objective-setting) and an observed client or colleague interaction (performance), followed by debriefing (self-reflection and feedback). Opportunities for communication coaching abound in the clinic setting, using role-play, video review, peer observation during appointments, or work shadowing. Research indicates that coaching in the clinic enhances veterinary professionals' communication skills and confidence, as well as elements of veterinarian and client satisfaction (Shaw et al. 2010, 2016; Cornell et al. 2019; Janke et al. 2022 and 2023) (Research Spotlights 9.1, 9.2, and 9.3).

Sidebar 9.2 Critical Tools for Communication Coaching

Delineate and apply key communication skills

Observe interactions

Foster self-reflection

Provide constructive feedback

Offer opportunities for practice

Host small group or one-on-one learning or training sessions

Source: Kurtz et al. (2005).

Research Spotlight 9.1

Communication Coaching Increases the Use of Effective Communication

In a study investigating the impact of communication coaching onsite in a veterinary practice, participants' use of communication skills differed after instruction. After a six-month training, veterinarians gathered significantly more client and environment data, and spent more time creating a partnership and relationship-building with clients. Clients in return provided more patient data and showed more empathy (Shaw et al. 2010).

In a similar study with a different veterinary practice, the use of communication skills again changed after a one-year training. Veterinarians used significantly fewer closed-ended inquiries, provided more client education, expressed more empathy, and spent more time focused on partnership building. Clients responded by providing more patient data and were engaged in more social conversation (Shaw et al. 2016).

In a third study with four veterinary practices, the use of client-centered communication skills increased after a 15-month intervention. Veterinarians elicited clients' agenda, expressed partnership, asked for client opinions, and invited clients to share more after training. Clients in turn asked lifestyle-social questions and provided more lifestyle-social information, and shared concern, optimism, reassurance, or encouragement with their veterinarian (Janke et al. 2023).

These findings demonstrate that communication is a learned skill that can be developed, and it is worth investing in communication training for the veterinary team.

Research Spotlight 9.2

Communication Coaching Enhances Client Satisfaction

An assessment of client satisfaction after veterinarians underwent a six-month communication skills training program revealed that clients felt significantly more involved and that clients felt the veterinarians expressed greater interest in their opinion following the training (Shaw et al. 2016). In a separate study of client satisfaction following a 15-month, in-practice communication training program, the odds of clients being completely satisfied were significantly higher after the communication skills intervention (Janke et al. 2022). These results demonstrate that communication training and coaching improve client satisfaction, which in turn benefits the veterinary practice.

Research Spotlight 9.3

Communication Coaching Enhances Veterinarian Satisfaction

In the study involving a six-month communication skills training program for veterinarians (Shaw et al. 2016), an evaluation of veterinarian satisfaction post-training showed that veterinarians perceived their clients as complaining significantly less and as being more personable and trusting. These findings highlight the professional benefits gained by veterinary team members from investing in communication skills training and coaching.

> **Sidebar 9.3   Coaching Communication Skills**
>
> **Elicit colleague's perspective**
>
> Open-ended inquiry
> Pause
> Reflective listening
> Chunk and check
>
> **Provide structure**
>
> Internal summary
> Signpost
> Contracts for next steps
>
> **Build relationships**
>
> Asking permission
> Partnership
> Empathy

In this chapter, we apply many of the communication skills introduced in the previous chapters to coaching colleagues (Sidebar 9.3). As coaches, we use these communication skills to elicit a colleague's perspective, structure coaching sessions, build a relationship, provide supportive feedback, and create a safe learning environment. We provide examples in two settings: a coaching session between the practice manager, Jenny Thu-Hong, and Dr. Alyssa Moss to work through recent client complaints; and a video-review session with Ms. Thu-Hong and a group of the practice's veterinary technicians.

Set the Scene

Colleague Scenario: In the first scenario, Dr. Alyssa Moss is an early-career associate veterinarian, who recently joined the practice. Unfortunately, within the first few months, she received a handful of client complaints. They boil down to struggles with time management and client communication. Clients are frustrated by long wait times and how Dr. Moss handles them. These grievances were brought to the attention of the practice manager, Jenny Thu-Hong, who reached out to Dr. Moss to provide support and coaching.

Team Scenario: In the second scenario, Ms. Thu-Hong schedules a coaching session with a group of veterinary technicians (Jan, Alexandra, and Nigel) to conduct video-review rounds.

Stepping into Jenny's shoes, self-reflect on:

1. How would I coach Dr. Moss with her time management and client communication struggles?
2. How would I conduct video review rounds with the team of veterinary technicians?

Attend to the Process of Communication Coaching

The process, or **how**, of being an effective coach is to use a partner communication style with colleagues; provide specific, detailed, balanced, relevant feedback; and conduct supportive and structured coaching sessions.

Communication Styles

The communication styles presented in Chapter 2 concerning communicating with clients – expert vs. partner – are an equally important consideration when coaching colleagues. The expert takes the lead, does most of the talking, and sets the agenda, while the partner seeks collaboration, mutual dialogue, and a shared agenda (see Figure 2.1 in Chapter 2). As with clients, it is common for us to default to the expert role; however, the partner style is most effective when coaching colleagues.

Our coaching style often reflects our personality traits, temperament, and character. We possess a natural communication style that feels most comfortable and a default style that we lean on when stressed. So do our colleagues. As a coach, we may need to flex, sometimes beyond our comfort zone, to use the partner style.

Expert

As a refresher, the expert style is when the veterinary professional drives the agenda as the expert-in-charge or expert-guide, and colleagues play a more passive role. This communication approach is referred to as the "talking head," symbolized by a **shot-put** (Barbour 2000; Kurtz et al. 2005). With a shot-put, the focus is on the delivery of information, and it may be challenging for colleagues to buy in, particularly when the information is not aligned with their perspective.

The expert role is common in veterinary practice and is misconstrued as coaching. The strength of the expert approach is that it offers clear, direct, and quick communication. This style exudes confidence, leads to decisive action, and moves agendas forward. It "gets things done" early on. However, it is difficult to achieve desired long-term results.

The challenge is that the expert prioritizes efficient one-sided decision-making over cooperative involvement and buy-in. Therefore, the expert's colleagues may feel steamrolled or pressured "to do as they are told." Because of the lack of opportunity to voice their thoughts, opinions, and beliefs, colleagues may not speak up if they think differently or feel an approach will not work for them; they may not be bought in to the approach or feel the support needed to carry it through.

Partner

In coaching, the veterinary professional plays the role of partner or facilitator, striving for mutual agreement with colleagues. This collaborative approach takes the form of a discussion, symbolized by a **Frisbee** (Barbour 2000; Kurtz et al. 2005), where the interaction is reciprocal. This approach values the exchange of information, invites engagement, and assists colleagues in navigating their own path forward in a supportive manner. During consensus-building, buy-in is favored over timely decision-making.

The upside of the partnership approach is the engaging dialogue that elicits feedback and then checks to ensure that both parties are moving forward together. This process provides space for colleagues' voices, thoughts, and concerns; we rely on our colleagues' expertise. This brainstorming approach may result in more creative and diverse solutions that align with our colleagues' needs and styles.

The downside is that a partnership approach can take longer. If structure is lacking in these conversations, it may be difficult to maintain momentum and direction, causing frustration and slowing progress. However, by taking the time up front, partners often save time in the long run by mitigating colleague resentment, dissatisfaction, and discontent.

As a coach, being a partner is the most effective way to help colleagues develop new skills. The partner style engages colleagues as equals. The colleague identifies their communication objectives and drives learning and growth. This empowering approach enhances colleague investment, buy-in, and commitment to change. Our colleague is in the driver's seat, and we – as the coach – are in the passenger's seat, providing support and avoiding backseat driving.

Coach Communication

The coaching approach uses a partner communication style. The coach is a facilitator whose specific intention is to assist in developing our colleagues' areas of opportunity as well as existing areas of strength. The coach uses questions to guide their colleagues' thought processes and assist them in identifying their own needs, skills, and motivations for change (Box 9.1). Therefore, during coaching, the colleague, rather than the coach, sets the direction, objectives, and expectations for the work.

Box 9.1 Guiding Questions for Coaching

What communication skill(s) would you like to focus on during this client (or colleague) interaction?
What are your thoughts about what it might have been like for your client (or colleague)?
What do you think attributed to the success or difficulty of this interaction?
How might you approach this situation differently next time around?
What is another way you might approach this conversation?
What has worked well for you in the past?
What other experiences can you draw from?
How will today's discussion change how you work with clients (or colleagues) in the future?
What changes might you implement based on this experience?
How can I support and mentor you in making these changes? <ask one at a time>

The coach's intention is to challenge their peers to grow professionally and take their skillset to the next level. An effective coach supports self-directed discovery and development in their peers (Adams and Kurtz 2012). The end goal is for the colleague to discover, with skillful guidance, the answer(s) for themselves.

The challenge is that not all colleagues want to grow and develop. Some may possess a fixed mindset and not be receptive to feedback or motivated to change; others may feel threatened. They may lack self-initiative, resourcefulness, or self-awareness and may not welcome specific instruction or external direction from others. This is where the coaching skills outlined in this chapter come into play to create safe, supportive, and constructive settings and diffuse feelings of vulnerability and resistance.

Provide Specific, Descriptive, Balanced, and Relevant Feedback

Feedback is information about the performance of a task used as a basis for changing behavior to achieve further growth and is paramount for personal and professional development (Brookhart 2017). Feedback is used to assess, educate, motivate, and align expectations for advancing skills. Frame and structure feedback encounters to prevent defensiveness and foster receptivity (Box 9.2). Feedback is in the hands of the deliverer, although how it is heard is in the ears, mind, and heart of the receiver.

Box 9.2 Structure a Feedback Encounter for Success

1. **Integrate feedback into everyday conversations.** Make it casual, routine, and commonplace rather than associated only with performance reviews.
   If you have a moment after you finish up, I'd love to chat about some client feedback. [asking permission]

2. **Start with colleague's self-assessment.** Invite your colleagues to share their thoughts to discover how the interaction went from their perspective, what they felt was effective, and how they might approach it differently or what they would like to change.
   Share with me how that interaction went for you. [open-ended inquiry]

3. **Be well-intentioned and empathetic.** Create a supportive setting for colleagues to be open and courageous and to take risks.
*I also **struggle** with pauses; it's **hard** for me to keep my mouth shut.* [empathy]

4. **Ask permission to offer feedback.** Place control in the receiver's hands: ask if they are ready to receive feedback and if not, offer to reschedule to another time.
***Would you be open to** discussing some recent feedback I received from Mrs. Mughrabi, who you saw on Monday?* [asking permission]

5. **Limit feedback to amounts that are useful and realistic.** Prioritize the most pertinent points and stay on-message. Keep feedback concise and succinct to enhance the possibility of the feedback being well-received, recalled, and put into practice.
Consider breaking your introduction down into greeting the client and pet, introducing yourself, clarifying your role, and then focusing on agenda-setting. [chunk]

6. **Check on how the feedback was received.** Remain sensitive to the recipient's reaction, and consider what next steps may be needed to promote learning.
What are your thoughts on this feedback? [check]

7. **Offer support and mentorship moving forward.** Be an available, accessible, approachable partner.
***How** can I support you in working on these skills?* [open-ended inquiry]
***What** steps would you like to take together to move forward?* [open-ended inquiry]
*I'm available around 2:00 p.m. **Would you like to** get together for some tea and brainstorm?* [asking permission]

Adapted from Hunter and Shaw (2018a).

When feedback is vague, blurred, or indirect, it may result in confusion or misunderstanding on the recipient's part. On the other hand, clear feedback sometimes seems too direct – even blunt – and, as a result, individuals may feel vulnerable or threatened or go on the defensive (Stone and Heen 2014). In this case, our well-meaning observations may be deflected and dismissed. When our feedback is specific, descriptive, balanced, focused on behavior, and limited in scope, it is more likely to be heard and incorporated (Box 9.3).

Box 9.3   How to Give Effective Feedback

Here are some suggestions for how to give effective feedback:

1. Deliver **descriptive and specific feedback** using chunk-and-check.
I saw that when you entered the exam room, you began with "So, when did the vomiting start?" and missed a chance to introduce yourself to Ms. Smith and clarify your role at the practice. [chunk] ***What** was happening for you at the beginning of the appointment?* [check]

2. Provide **balanced feedback** that includes areas of strength and future opportunities, including suggestions of something to try in the future.
The client mentioned they appreciated the time you took to put her dog at ease before conducting your physical exam. [area of strength] *You might also take a moment to make the client*

(Continued)

Box 9.3 (Continued)

more comfortable by introducing yourself and your role at the practice at the beginning of the interaction. [future opportunity and suggestion]

3. **Link feedback to outcomes**, such as "put her dog at ease" in the previous example. *Getting the visit off to the right start **puts clients and their pets at ease**, builds **rapport**, and forms a **friendly, trusting basis** for your **relationship** with the client.*

4. **Use *and* in place of *but*** to reinforce, rather than detract from, the positive feedback provided. A *but* in a sentence negates everything said up to that point and may trigger defensiveness. *The attention to detail with Bruno's chart helped when I reviewed his case. **And** providing the same level of detail with your care instructions in discharge statements could benefit our clients and the continuity of care between doctors.*

5. **Focus on behaviors** rather than personality traits. Emphasize actions and behaviors to underscore that the opportunity lies in what an individual does or does not do, not in who they are. *I liked how you guided Mr. Aragon, who was visibly crying, into an examination room to continue your discussion. **How** might that approach work with clients who are becoming agitated or upset?* [open-ended inquiry] *In particular, I was thinking about Mrs. Mughrabi, who was really frustrated about having to wait.*

6. **Offer suggestions, not directives** (e.g. *what if, I wonder, could this work, you might try*, or *something to consider*). Share information in a way that respects the receiver and empowers them. *You need to, you must*, and *you should* sound authoritative and may be interpreted as advice-giving, prescriptive, evaluative, or judgmental. *One suggestion to slow yourself down: **you might** take a deep breath before entering the exam room, so you're ready to give the client your full attention.* [chunk] *What are your thoughts?* [check]

7. Encourage colleagues to **forward plan** and take responsibility for their learning. *Given our conversation, how would you like to address the next frustrated client you encounter?* [open-ended inquiry]

Adapted from Kurtz et al. (2005) and Hunter and Shaw (2018a).

Receive Feedback with an Open Mind

As important as how we deliver feedback is how we receive it. One thing that rouses our defense mechanisms is when we perceive feedback as an evaluation or criticism instead of an opportunity for growth. To develop an awareness of these reactions, it is instructive to ask ourselves: do we filter feedback through the lens of a **fixed** or a **growth** mindset (Dweck 2016)? A person with a more fixed mindset reasons that traits and abilities are stagnant and set in stone ("I am who I am, and nothing you say is going to change that"). On the other hand, a person with a growth mindset understands that characteristics and capacities are constantly in flux, adapting, and progressing ("I am constantly growing, learning, and embracing opportunities for change").

So, in receiving feedback, what is absorbed and what is deflected is based on our mindset (Dweck 2016). To a colleague with a fixed mindset, who perceives feedback as a threat to self, a workplace that routinely incorporates coaching may feel hostile; this person may go on the defensive, and retreat. However, adopting and nurturing a growth mentality reframes deficits into opportunities for development and setbacks into challenges to tackle. Creating a clinic culture where coaching is routine, and feedback is viewed from a growth perspective, is beneficial for turning moments of breakdown into opportunities and occasions to learn. In this nonjudgmental context, feedback is often sought out versus repelled by others.

Being receptive to feedback is a delicate dance of determining what was heard and what was meant (Stone and Heen 2014). An effective coach elicits responses, reactions, and viewpoints of others to explore how the feedback was received and considers how different perspectives could be helpful. In response, colleagues shift from flight-or-fight to an open-minded, curious, and interested stance (Box 9.4).

Box 9.4   How to Receive Feedback

1. **Ask clarifying questions** to prevent misinterpretation.
   So, because I was in a hurry at the beginning of the visit, Mrs. Mughrabi thought that I didn't care about her and Beau's long wait. [reflective listening] *Oh, okay. That's a helpful observation! So, how could I handle that differently?* [open-ended inquiry]

2. **Request specific examples** to clarify, assimilate, and create a clearer picture for moving forward.
   Would you give me an example, so I can get a better understanding of what you mean? [asking permission]
   In what other scenarios do you see this happening? [open-ended inquiry]

3. **Seek additional perspectives**; request further observation, coaching, and feedback to put change into practice and promote professional growth.
   Would you mind observing my next appointment for these behaviors? [asking permission]
   What do you suggest I do differently? [open-ended inquiry]

4. **Plan forward**. Come up with ideas and give them a try "live" to see how they work in a role-play scenario or with a client in the examination room.
   I'd like to try introducing myself formally and apologizing for running late. Then offer partnership up front, ask the client's permission to move forward, and see how that works.

Adapted from Hunter and Shaw (2018b) and Stone and Heen (2014).

Learn to Be a Communication Coach

To be an effective coach, consider the various contexts and settings in which coaching occurs, prepare colleagues ahead of time, and use a systematic coaching process to balance providing support and encouraging colleagues to challenge themselves.

Take into Account Various Coaching Contexts

Coaching can be used by and with individuals in every practice role (veterinarian, hospital manager, veterinary technician, and assistant), and it is effective for diverse purposes and contexts (e.g. mentoring, onboarding, and performance reviews). In addition, various settings within the veterinary hospital are well-suited for coaching (e.g. front desk, examination room, treatment room, office, and staff lounge).

Consider Coaching Levels of Difficulty

Coaching scenarios fall into beginner, intermediate, and advanced levels (Sidebar 9.4). Take into consideration the context and nature of the conversation, the seriousness of the topic, the potential consequences, and the people involved. As a developing coach, progress from easier, predictable, structured one-on-one coaching scenarios to more challenging free-form group interactions. Move from straightforward training or mentoring situations to conducting performance reviews or addressing complaints, in which conflict is more likely to arise. Confidence and competence will grow with practice and over time as the coaching process falls into place.

Sidebar 9.4   Coaching Levels of Difficulty

Beginner Coach

Guidance: Offer this when a colleague approaches for advice and brainstorming.
Video review and reflection one-on-one: Side by side, review a videorecording of a client or colleague interaction.
Role-play one-on-one: Use a case-based scenario to role-play an interaction and practice communication skills with one individual.

Intermediate Coach

Orientation and onboarding – Prepare a new team member for their role in the practice, including discussion and demonstration of job responsibilities and tasks.
Ongoing personnel training: Help a colleague with continual skill development or expansion of job responsibilities and tasks.
Mentoring sessions: Assist with a colleague's professional development to take tasks to the next skill level or obtain a promotion.
Role-play in a small group: Use a case-based scenario to role-play an interaction and practice communication skills within a small group.
Video review and reflection in a small group: Review a videorecording of a client or colleague interaction with a gathering of colleagues.
Team meetings: Conduct regular small-group or large, entire-practice meetings.

Advanced Coach

In-the-moment coaching: Provide this through spontaneous observation or job shadowing.
Performance reviews: Formally or informally evaluate job performance on a regular and annual basis.
Client and team concerns: Address concerns as they arise, and brainstorm solutions moving forward.

Choose an Appropriate Setting for Coaching

A coaching session may be formalized and scheduled, such as for mentoring, training, or performance review. Or it may be informal, spontaneous, and in-the-moment when a learning opportunity arises on the spot from observing a client or colleague interaction (Box 9.5). In-the-moment is an advanced coaching practice and requires keen observation, appropriate timing and place, receptivity to learning, and a trusting practice culture.

Box 9.5   Look for In-the-Moment Communication Coaching Opportunities

Client service coordinators: Observe client check-ins or check-outs at the front desk or listen in on live or recorded telephone conversations with clients.

Veterinary assistants: Observe setting up appointments for clients in the examination room or colleague-colleague interactions in the treatment room.

Veterinary technicians: Observe agenda-setting and information-gathering with clients in the examination room or colleague-colleague interactions in the treatment room.

Veterinarians: Observe client interactions in the examination room or colleague-colleague interactions in the treatment room.

Practice managers: Observe colleague-colleague interactions during individual discussions, small group interactions, or staff meetings.

Practice owners: Observe client interactions in the examination room and colleague-colleague interactions during individual discussions, small group interactions, or staff meetings.

The material for communication-skills coaching sessions comes from several sources: an observed or video-recorded client or colleague interaction, a role-play exercise, or a formal simulation. The practice setting is ripe for collecting live examples of client and colleague interactions in various settings with multiple players. The key to effective role-playing is authentic re-creation based on a real-life client or colleague interaction. Simulation using professional actor-educators (simulated clients) is primarily reserved for educational settings (veterinary communication curricula or continuing education). Such simulations are often reenactments of case-based scenarios in a room equipped for video recording with simulated clients, a trained coach, and a small group of colleagues.

Use Role-Play to Provide Coaching Opportunities

Role-play was introduced as an activity in previous chapters (Chapters 3 and 7). Although it is a powerful learning technique, role-play is fraught with comedic, silly, yet fun dramatizations. The key is to base the role-play on a real client or colleague scenario. The fact that it really happened and is grounded in true (not fictitious) events makes for a meaningful interaction.

There are two ways to create an authentic role-play interaction. The first is to use a recent client or colleague interaction and ask the individual who was originally involved in the interaction to step into the role of mock client or colleague and invite another colleague to practice a skill with the "simulated client or colleague". In the client or colleague role, the individual replies as they perceive the client or colleague would, based on their previous interaction. This person is uniquely positioned to share insights into how they think the original client or colleague may respond.

Another way to make a role-play exercise genuine is to ask a colleague to portray themselves as a client or colleague (Hunter and Shaw 2016). For example, ask a colleague to reflect on a time when they brought their own pet to a veterinarian or to think about a colleague interaction. Then reconstruct the scenario; where the colleague portrays what they were feeling, thinking, and experiencing at that time. The colleague is in a prime position to share perceptions of what it was like for them, how the situation was handled, what met their needs, and what they might like done differently.

Prepare the Team for Coaching

To prepare the team for communication coaching, introduce and define the concept of coaching and clearly elucidate the why (e.g. purpose, expectations, and goals) behind it. Address individual benefits as well as intended outcomes for the practice, veterinary team, clients, and patients.

Ask the team what they would like to gain from communication coaching and identify specifically what they hope to learn. Use the structure of this book to shape coaching interactions based on the steps of the clinical interview and incorporate the 20 communication skills presented. A shared learning culture enhances the efficacy of skill acquisition when everyone is talking about and working on a similar set of communication skills.

Being observed and coached is nerve-wracking for individuals, so take time to elicit the veterinary team's concerns, address their questions, and invite suggestions. Brainstorm how to balance comfort (being supported) with challenge (being stretched outside your comfort zone to try new skills). Identify group guidelines to create a safe and supportive environment to grow and learn (Box 9.6). These are behavioral norms defined by the team; they promote a comfortable learning environment. To pave the way, identify willing volunteers to be coached first, to serve as role models and lead by example.

Box 9.6   Examples of Small-Group Guidelines

Work with the team to identify group guidelines to ensure safety and supportiveness. The following are some sample phrases to get started. Establish an initial list, and then revisit it each coaching session. Remind each other of the commitment and modify or adapt as needed:

Confidentiality: *What happens here stays here and will not be shared or discussed with others.*

Listen: *Embrace silence so that everyone can share.*

Safety: *With our feedback, we will work together to create a safe space, support each other, and take a nonjudgmental stance.*

Practice: *The purpose of this role-play is to experiment, try out new skills, take a different approach, and allow each of us to grow.*

Challenge: *We will stretch outside our comfort zones to try new things. This may mean embracing the awkward, taking risks, and being courageous – this is where learning happens.*

Growth: *This activity is intended for growth and professional development through self-awareness, skill-honing, and objective-setting.*

Formative: *This is a continuing education exercise and will not be part of evaluating your job performance.*

Balance: *We will provide support and encourage each other to challenge ourselves.*

Diversity: *We will be embracing differences, as there are multiple right ways to communicate.*

Ascribe to Coaching Philosophies

After years of training and working with coaches, we developed mantras that encapsulate key coaching principles in a series of simple statements. We provide litmus tests as a self-test to differentiate coaching versus leading. These guidelines boil down to asking lots of reflective, open-ended inquiries, practicing silence, keeping our own thoughts at bay, and allowing colleagues to come up with next steps:

1. **Meet colleague(s) where they are.**
   The litmus test is to balance the coach's agenda with the colleague's; ask, "Whose agenda is it?" We often envision where our colleague could go or what they could do. However, against our intuition, the more efficacious path to get there is to take a step back to ascertain our

colleague's perspective, elicit their ideas of their next move, or brainstorm with them potential routes to take. A colleague may not be progressing in their skill development as quickly as we expect or would like; however, they are growing leaps and bounds for themselves. This means patiently pacing with them and providing kudos on strides made and support to reach the next level. You might ask:

> **What** *would you like to achieve?* [open-ended inquiry]
> **How** *might you get there?* [open-ended inquiry]
> **What** *might you say or do?* [open-ended inquiry]

2. **Let colleague(s) do the work.**
   The litmus test is to check the coach's level of involvement; ask, "Who is doing all the work?" or "Who is doing all the talking?" The ideal answer is *My colleague*. If it is not, then you are not coaching; you are directing or leading. It is tempting to tell colleagues what to do. After all, coaches possess mounds of knowledge and experience and a strong and well-intentioned desire to help. However, people learn more when supported than when told what to do. You might ask:

> **What** *are your ideas for going forward?* [open-ended inquiry]
> **How** *do you think it may be received?* [open-ended inquiry]
> **What** *would be another approach?* [open-ended inquiry]

3. **Promote self-discovery by asking versus telling.**
   The litmus test is catching advice-giving; ask, "Whose idea was it in the end?" Instead of giving tips, suggestions, or answers, ask more open-ended inquiries, do more listening, and get comfortable with silence. The challenge with giving advice is that a colleague becomes reliant on receiving direction from others in lieu of becoming self-reliant, resourceful and taking initiative. By promoting self-discovery, you equip the team with problem-solving skills and empower them to find solutions on their own. This greater autonomy reduces the need for micro-management and frees time for higher-level leadership responsibilities. You might ask:

> **How** *do you think we can approach this situation?* [open-ended inquiry]
> **What** *would you do in this circumstance?* [open-ended inquiry]
> **What** *would be your first step or statement?* [open-ended inquiry]

Implement a Coaching Model

The coaching model provides a user-friendly script for all the players in a coaching session. Using this stepwise process introduces structure and supports collegial relationships. Follow all or some of the steps in the model, depending on the type of coaching activity. As coach, we are challenged to role-model the communication skills for our colleagues.

The process guides the coach to stay on track, provides consistency, and ensures that items are not missed. The framework provides a reliable roadmap to set expectations, create a safe and supportive learning environment, and reduce uncertainty. Even our most seasoned communication coaches stick to the coaching steps and advise new coaches, when in doubt, to trust the coaching process. One outline is fine-tuned for coaching one-on-one (Box 9.7), and the other is tailored to working with small groups or teams (Box 9.8).

Box 9.7   One-on-One Coaching

One-on-one coaching provides a scenario for colleagues to focus on and practice communication skills and an opportunity for the coach to observe and provide constructive feedback. Follow along with the **Coaching Process Card** (Appendix B):

1. **Prepare to coach.**
   a. Take a minute to inhale deeply and get grounded before going into the coaching session, to bring a relaxed stance, calm demeanor, and full presence to the interaction.
   b. Review the work schedule or appointment bookings to ensure that no urgent/emergent patients arrived and that the timing is good.
   c. Gather up tools, such as a clipboard, pen, and paper for notetaking, the **20 Communication Skills** (Appendix A) definitions and examples, and the **Communication Skills Checklist** (Appendix C) to stay on track.

2. **Open the session.**
   When in a hurry, it is easy to skip critical steps; if they are neglected, the session loses its efficacy. So, before starting, review this outline, and then engage in the following ways:
   a. Establish rapport.
      How are you doing, Dr. Moss? [open-ended inquiry]
   b. Demonstrate interest and concern
      I appreciate you taking the time to work together. [partnership]
   c. Review the purpose of the interaction/appointment.
      Dr. Moss, this is an opportunity for us to work together on some of the communication challenges you are experiencing. [chunk] *What are your thoughts coming into this?* [check]
   d. Establish a safe, supportive, and confidential atmosphere.
      *I anticipate that we're going to learn a lot from **each other**.* [partnership]
      *Our work **together** is confidential and will not be shared with anyone else, working in the practice or otherwise.* [partnership]
   e. Outline the session steps:
      ***Let's start by** talking about your communication objectives.* [signpost]
      ***Then** I will observe your appointment* [signpost]
      ***Afterward**, we'll debrief, starting with your impressions, and **then** I'll share some observations and thoughts for consideration.* [signpost]
      Finally, we'll end by identifying your objectives moving forward. [signpost]
      How does that sound to you? [open-ended inquiry]

3. **Prep for the interaction/appointment.**
   a. Review the interviewer's communication objectives.
      *Dr. Moss, **what** specific communication skills would you like to work on?* [open-ended inquiry]
      ***What** led you to choose those skills?* [open-ended inquiry]
      ***You mentioned** focusing on your introduction.* [reflective listening] ***What** else?* [open-ended inquiry]
      ***What** do you see as your strengths?* [open-ended inquiry]
      ***What** may be a stretch for you?* [open-ended inquiry]

    b. Brainstorm communication skills and objectives.
       __What__ would that sound like? [open-ended inquiry]
       __What__ might that look like? [open-ended inquiry]
       __How__ might you say that? [open-ended inquiry]
       __How__ might you make it your own? [open-ended inquiry]

    c. Plan for feedback.
       __What__ specifically would you like me to look for? [open-ended inquiry]
       __How__ can I help you with that? [open-ended inquiry]
       __Would you__ like me to video-record the appointment? [asking permission]
       __What__ else do you need to do to prepare for this appointment? [open-ended inquiry]

4. **Observe the interaction.**

    a. Introduce yourself to the client(s) or colleague(s) and explain your role as an observer to coach your colleague on their communication skills. Request the client's or colleague's consent to observe and/or video-record the appointment or meeting. This is an important step to put clients at ease and not jeopardize their trust in the veterinary professional's medical training, expertise, and authority.
       Mrs. Kovak, I'm Jenny Thu-Hong, the practice manager. Dr. Moss asked me to observe this appointment and give her feedback on her communication skills. As a practice, we're working on communication so we can take even better care of you and Slinky.
       __Would it be all right__ if I observed and/or video-recorded today's appointment and jotted some notes? [asking permission] *I'll share my notes with Dr. Moss, and no one else, after the appointment. You and Slinky will still receive our best care.*

    b. Note examples of communication objectives demonstrated. Record specific examples (verbatim quotes or phrases and nonverbal descriptions) of the communication skills used most effectively during the interaction.

    c. Recognize growth opportunities to use additional communication skills, identifying specific client phrases or nonverbal behaviors from the interaction that highlight missed opportunities.

5. **Debrief the interaction/appointment.**

    a. Start with your colleague's self-assessment. To elicit their feedback, use open-ended inquiries such as these:
       Dr. Moss, __how__ did that go for you? [open-ended inquiry]
       __How__ did your identified communication skill objectives work for you? [open-ended inquiry]
       __What__ was challenging for you? [open-ended inquiry]
       __What__ would you do differently next time? [open-ended inquiry]

    b. Create an opportunity to rewind and role-play.
       __What__ would it sound like if you could do that over again? [open-ended inquiry]
       __Would__ you like to practice that with me? [asking permission]

    c. Ask permission to provide feedback.
       Dr. Moss, __could I__ share some thoughts on that? [asking permission]
       __Would you__ be open to hearing what I noticed? [asking permission]

(Continued)

Box 9.7 (Continued)

---

    d. Share feedback (Boxes 9.2 and 9.3).

       Dr. Moss, I liked how you handled running late. I saw you take a deep breath, formally introduce yourself, clarify your role, and greet Mrs. Kovak with a smile, which appeared to put both of you at ease. You offered partnership, "I am here now for you and Slinky." I saw Mrs. Kovak exhale and smile, and her shoulders visibly relaxed. [chunk] ***What*** *was that exchange like for you?* [check]

       Later in the interview, I saw her break eye contact and lean back in her chair when you talked about the need for anesthesia. [chunk] ***What*** *are your thoughts?* [check]
       What *could you say or do when Mrs. Kovak withdrew?* [open-ended inquiry]
       When you asked, "What concerns you most about this procedure?" you learned that Mrs. Kovak was fearful of anesthesia. [chunk] ***What*** *might be your next move?* [check]
       I heard Mrs. Kovak say that she'd had a previous bad experience with anesthesia with another dog. [chunk] ***What*** *did you hear?* [check]
       How *might you invite her to share more about her concern with anesthesia?* [open-ended inquiry]

    e. Create another opportunity to rewind and role-play
       How *would you phrase that differently?* [open-ended inquiry]
       Would you *like to try that out with me?* [asking permission]
       How *did that approach work for you?* [open-ended inquiry]

  6. **Close the session, and identify lessons learned and next steps.**
       What *is your takeaway from this client interaction?* [open-ended inquiry]
       What *communication strengths will you take to your next client interaction?* [open-ended inquiry]
       What *are you hoping to do differently in your next client interaction?* [open-ended inquiry]

       It seems like *you're feeling more solid about making introductions that set the tone for a productive appointment. Your next communication objective is to elicit the client's perspective to understand where they are coming from, using open-ended inquiry more and then offering partnership statements to indicate that you would like to support them.* [summary]
       What *would you like to add?* [open-ended inquiry]
       Okay, we have a plan*: You're going to ask Julie, your veterinary technician, to observe these skills and provide feedback during your appointments for the next two weeks. Then we'll set up another coaching session.* [contracts for next steps]
       How *else can I support you?* [final check]

Adapted from Kurtz et al. (2005).

Box 9.8 Small-Group Coaching

Coaching with a small group allows for more interactivity, experimentation, and dynamism, bringing in everyone's perspectives and ideas. The previous one-on-one coaching steps apply; add the following steps to conduct a small group coaching session. Follow along with the **Coaching Process Card** (Appendix B):

1. **Open the session.** Check in with everyone before proceeding.
    *On a scale from **1 to 10**, with 1 being relaxed and 10 being anxious, how are you coming into today's session?* [closed-ended inquiry]

*What **adjective** would you use to describe how you are feeling about today's training?* [closed-ended inquiry]

2. **Prep the interaction/appointment.** Incorporate the whole group in brainstorming communication approaches.
   ***Let's** create a list of examples for each of Alexandra's communication skill objectives to set her up for success.* [signpost]
   ***What** suggested phrases would you offer?* [open-ended inquiry]
   ***What** would you say in this scenario?* [open-ended inquiry]
   ***How** do you make that your own?* [open-ended inquiry]

3. **Observe the simulated or recorded interaction.** Assign each individual one of their colleague's communication skill objectives to watch for and record feedback on.
   ***Who** would like to watch for (communication skill)?* [closed-ended inquiry]
   ***Who** is also working on (communication skill)?* [closed-ended inquiry]

4. **Debrief the interaction/appointment.** Integrate the whole group in debriefing the session.
   ***We'll start** with your self-assessment, Alexandra, then we'll hear from your peers, and finally, I will offer coach feedback.* [signpost]
   *Alexandra, first, **how** did that go for you?* [open-ended inquiry]
   ***Let's start** with <communication skill> – who was observing that?* [closed-ended inquiry]
   ***What** did you see?* [open-ended inquiry]
   ***What** might you say in this circumstance?* [open-ended inquiry]
   ***Let's** try it out <new role-play>.* [signpost]
   ***How** did that approach work for you? <debrief the new role-play>* [open-ended inquiry]

5. **Close, and identify lessons learned and next steps.**
   ***Let's** go around the group and each share an "aha" moment from the group session.* [signpost]
   ***What** is your take-home lesson or idea?* [open-ended inquiry]
   ***What** are you walking away with?* [open-ended inquiry]

   ***You shared three key approaches** – apologizing, offering partnership, and providing assurances that the client and pet will receive the care they deserve – for diffusing frustrated clients.* [summary] ***What** else would you add to the list?* [open-ended inquiry]
   ***We agreed to** individually focus on a key skill for the next week and to report on our strengths and opportunities at our next weekly technicians' meeting.* [contracts for next steps]
   ***How** else can I help you address these challenges?* [final check]

Adapted from Kurtz et al. (2005).

Offer Opportunities to Practice

One of the greatest advantages of role-play and simulation is the ability to start, stop, and "rewind" the interaction at any point in time. Rewinds are a coaching technique that offers individuals a "do-over" or an opportunity to try something new. They are often just one or two sentences, enough of an exchange to try a skill and see how the individual responds. There are multiple places to use the rewind strategy during a coaching session (Box 9.9). Rewinds are one of the coach's most effective tools, as they present a short, low-stakes chance to try it out, experiment, and see the response.

Box 9.9 Opportunities to Rewind

Rewinds are used in multiple places during a role-play or simulation to optimize learning:

In the middle of the interaction during a pause: When the conversation did not proceed as intended, it is a "do-over" moment to try another approach and see how it works.
Would you *like to rewind and try a different approach?* [asking permission]
What *would you like to do differently this time?* [open-ended inquiry]

During debriefing: Give everyone a chance to practice the communication skills and "give it a try."
What *would you say to use (communication skill) in this interaction?* [open-ended inquiry]
Where *would you like to resume the conversation to give it a try?* [closed-ended inquiry]

Post-feedback: Empower the primary learner to take charge of their learning process by choosing and trying out a piece of feedback they received.
Of the suggestions provided, ***what*** *would you like to try?* [open-ended inquiry]

During a coaching session, use rewinds to:

1. Present a colleague who struggled with a specific communication skill another chance to practice and build confidence and competence.
2. Offer an opportunity for success when the conversation did not go as the colleague wanted the first time. This is particularly fulfilling when a previous interaction did not go well, and a colleague regains a sense of accomplishment.
3. Take pressure off the colleague in the hot seat by temporarily redirecting the focus of learning to other members of the group. Someone else steps in to try a communication skill.
4. Shift the debriefing conversation from a feedback lecture to an engaging round of experimentation and practice. It prevents colleagues from being the critic on the sideline and provides an opportunity to step into the ring and try it themselves.
5. Give nervous colleagues a chance to warm up their communication skills in a brief, low-risk interaction. Because rewinds are short and simple, they lessen the anxiety of being responsible for a more involved interaction.

Attend to the Content of Communication Coaching

The content, or **what**, of how to be an effective coach is to view colleagues as experts and elicit their perspectives.

View Colleagues as Experts

The veterinary team is composed commonly of veterinarians, veterinary technicians, veterinary assistants, client-service coordinators or representatives, practice managers, and owners. Each member possesses specialized clinical, technical, professional, organizational, and interpersonal expertise. So, everyone is an expert in their own area, with complementary and integrated skillsets dovetailing with those of the rest of the team (Kinnison et al. 2014). When we capitalize on the team's wealth of knowledge and experiences, more creative solutions come to fruition than would come solely from ourselves alone. A cohesive whole is better than the sum of individual parts.

As a coach, we respect our colleagues' expertise, break down hierarchical structures and communication barriers, and invite contributions from every team member (Kinnison et al. 2014). It is a balancing act between personal development and team performance. We support individual advancement and contributions, investing in their professional development and delegating tasks within their capabilities. And at the same time, we create a coordinated team through structured communication, teamwork, and establishing shared goals. The results are worth it: enhanced individual engagement (Moore et al. 2014, Pizzolon et al. 2019), more efficient team performance, better service of clients and patients, and greater practice productivity (Kinnison et al. 2014) (Research Spotlight 9.4).

Research Spotlight 9.4

Individual Engagement Promotes Job Satisfaction

Two survey studies of veterinary team members investigated the relationship between team effectiveness and job satisfaction. Both found that individual engagement increased job satisfaction (Moore et al. 2014; Pizzolon et al. 2019). Individual engagement results from being recognized as a valuable member of the team, assigned responsibilities within the designated role, and appreciated for work contributions. These results highlight the importance of prizing each team member's contributions as well as empowering them in their job, which leads to enhanced job satisfaction.

Elicit Colleague's Perspective

One of the *Seven Habits of Highly Effective Leaders* is first to seek to understand and then to be understood (Covey 2004). This entails starting the coaching conversation with eliciting our colleague's perspective, including their impressions, feelings, and concerns about a situation. Then explore their objectives, expectations, priorities, ideas, and beliefs; what may be affecting their life and work; their learning style; and relevant knowledge, experiences, and background (see Chapter 4). Although it may not be possible to touch on all these facets in every coaching discussion, asking questions and gaining insight into our colleagues' perspective not only engages and empowers them but also prepares us for a more informed and deliberate coaching and feedback conversation.

Undoubtedly there will be times when we do not see eye to eye with our colleagues. In these moments of difference, we show our support by acknowledging a colleague's standpoint without necessarily agreeing with it. This nonjudgmental stance allows us to agree to disagree and maintain respect at the same time. A critical component of the coaching dynamic is that we do not want our colleagues to feel criticized, judged, or cornered into a defensive position. With acknowledgment, colleagues feel heard and respected; it supports their outlook in a way that begins to create common ground through shared understanding.

Commonly Asked Questions Related to Communication Coaching

What If My Colleague Becomes Defensive?

It takes courage to participate in a coaching session. Initially, some colleagues may feel vulnerable and become either defensive or emotional during the coaching session. Supporting colleagues calls for a balance of providing compassionate support while holding up expectations.

The more we employ coaching in our practice, the more our colleagues will adapt and accept it as part of their professional development. Consistency in coaching and modeling communication skills builds safety for our colleagues; they know what to expect, reducing uncertainty. It is helpful to create a forum for colleagues to share their experiences and feelings, especially at first, to ease anxiety and pave the path forward.

A guarded response is most frequently seen in individuals with a fixed mindset, where being coached feels like being evaluated or criticized. These team members may make excuses for not participating, delay scheduling their coaching session, or avoid it altogether. When receiving feedback, they may blame others instead of taking responsibility for their own actions. Be patient and present, keep pace with them, and seek to understand their perspective.

There are two potential paths for moving forward with a defensive colleague. The first is patience and persistence; meet them where they are, and with trust and rapport building, they may slowly turn the corner. The second is to make the call to dismiss the individual from the practice, depending on the practice culture. If embracing a growth mindset and being receptive to feedback are core practice values, this individual might not be a good fit for the practice team.

What If My Colleague Cries?

Often, there are underlying reasons why colleagues may turn to tears during communication training. Be mindful of not taking crying personally or shutting down in response. Weeping or tearing up in front of others may be an empathetic response to the clinical scenario itself or a colleague's response to the client's and/or patient's situation. Sometimes crying is the release of a pressure valve – an outlet for the stress of being observed or of work or home life. In addition, a colleague who cries may feel unsafe, evaluated, or judged, indicating the need for more support in future coaching sessions. Or the colleague who struggles with perfectionism may possess a strong inner critic.

Ask colleagues beforehand how they would like to receive feedback; they know themselves well. For some, receiving feedback triggers memories of parents, teachers, or coaches who provided harsh, critical, or judgmental feedback. Some individuals respond well to direct feedback (Nerf ball to the side of the head), while others need soft guidance (feather tickle to their face). Explore their perspective, empathize with their viewpoint and vulnerability, and identify how to best support them (Box 9.10).

Box 9.10   Supporting Colleagues During Challenging Moments

The following are some tips on how to support an emotional colleague during a coaching session:

1. Take a minute to pause and allow them to catch their breath, go to the bathroom, or grab a drink of water, as this allows the time that is often needed to get back on track.
   Take your time. *I'm here for you.* [partnership]
   Would you *like a drink of water or a cup of tea?* [asking permission]
   Shall we *hear your colleagues' thoughts and come back to you?* [asking permission]

2. Ask permission to see if they are ready to move forward. If they say "no," then reschedule the feedback session for another time.
   Are you *ready to talk about your client interaction?* [asking permission]
   Would you *like to share what's going on?* [asking permission]
   Would you *feel more comfortable if we took our conversation to another room?* [asking permission]

Would you *like to take a walk with me?* [asking permission]
Would you *like to take some time to reflect and process, and then reschedule our debriefing?* [asking permission]

3. Use open-ended inquiry to check in and seek colleague's perspective up front.
   How *are you doing?* [open-ended inquiry]
   What *was that like for you?* [open-ended inquiry]

4. Empathize with their viewpoint to validate their feelings.
   *I sense your **hesitation** with role-play and appreciate you giving this a chance.* [empathy]
   *It's **hard**, working with emotional clients. Thanks for stepping up to the plate.* [empathy]
   *It can be **nerve-wracking** to feel like you're being watched, even without being judged.* [empathy]
   *I appreciate that was a **challenging** interaction, especially when the client ramped up in frustration.* [empathy]

5. Capitalize on your colleague's communication strengths.
   I saw that empathy and open-ended inquiry are areas of strength for you. [chunk] ***What** are your thoughts?* [check]

6. Focus on the outcomes to highlight what was accomplished in the interaction.
   How *did the client respond to your empathy statements?* [open-ended inquiry]
   What *information did you glean from your open-ended inquiries?* [open-ended inquiry]

7. Set clear expectations.
   *We can reschedule this session so you can receive feedback from your colleagues later. **What** can I do to support you now?* [open-ended inquiry]

Colleague Scenario

Set the Scene: Jenny Thu-Hong, practice manager, requests a coaching session with Dr. Alyssa Moss, a new associate veterinarian at the practice, to discuss recent client complaints about time management and client communication.

JENNY: *Dr. Moss, **would you have a moment** for me to share with you some recent feedback I received from a few clients?* [asking permission]

DR. MOSS: *Sure! The clients have been great to work with!*

JENNY: ***Agreed**: for the most part, our clients really enjoy working with you.* [reflective listening] ***And there've been a few situations**, over the past couple of days, in which clients left the practice feeling dissatisfied.* [signpost – warning shot]

DR. MOSS: *Who was it? I bet it was the day we were slammed with emergencies. There's nothing I could've done about that.*

JENNY: ***Yes**, that's when most of the concerns came in.* [reflective listening] *I'm curious about **your perspective**.* [signpost] ***Let's** find a quiet place to talk about what happened and brainstorm **together** about how to handle these situations in the future.* [partnership]

DR. MOSS: *What did they say about me?*

JENNY: ***Before*** *discussing the specific details of what was shared by the clients, I am going to suggest we take a* ***step back****.* [signpost] *It sounds like it was a* ***stressful*** *day with many emergencies.* [empathy] ***Fill*** *me in.* [open-ended inquiry]

DR. MOSS: *It was a stressful day! I ran from one appointment to the next. There were a couple of critical patients. There were also several appointment slots double-booked. I didn't even have time to go to the bathroom or grab lunch.*

JENNY: *Oh, wow, that is* ***rough****!* [empathy] ***I didn't realize*** *that you were double-booked on top of worrisome cases.* [reflective listening] *With all that* ***pressure*** *and* ***stress,*** [empathy] ***How*** *did your appointments go?* [open-ended inquiry]

DR. MOSS: *Well, I triaged the most concerning patients and saw them first, which, of course, left the other clients waiting and wondering why I wasn't seeing their pets. Some of them were irritated by the time I met them in the examination room.*

Jenny: ***Yeah****, the clients I heard from were frustrated by the wait and not knowing when they'd be seen.* [reflective listening] ***Wha****t are some approaches* ***we*** *might try as a team* [partnership] *when the schedule gets chaotic?* [open-ended inquiry]

DR. MOSS: *I don't know. What recommendations do you have?* [open-ended inquiry]

JENNY: ***Before*** *jumping to solutions,* [signpost] *and to get a better idea of how I can help,* ***I'm wondering if*** *I can observe some of your appointments.* [asking permission]

Team Scenario

Set the Scene: Jenny Thu-Hong, practice manager and communication coach, hosts a video review session with Jan, Alexandra, and Nigel, members of the veterinary technician team. Jan volunteers to present a recent interaction with a client and their new baby. After Jan self-reflects, Jenny works with Alexandra and Nigel to present specific, descriptive, balanced, and relevant feedback.

JENNY: *Thanks, Jan, for offering to go first and presenting your video.* ***Share*** *with us your thoughts after seeing it again* [open-ended inquiry]

JAN: *I hate hearing my voice on video.*

JENNY: *It's* ***strange*** *to hear yourself, and we never sound like we imagine.* [empathy] *So,* ***diving in,*** [signpost] *you were working on open-ended inquiry, pause, and empathy.* [reflective listening]

JAN: *Well, the first thing I noticed was that I didn't know how to relate to the client's new baby.*

JENNY: *It can be* ***tough*** *to address something that seems personal,* [empathy] *and I appreciate your thoughtful reflection. I anticipate the group has* ***suggestions****.* [signpost] ***Are you open to*** *hearing their feedback?* [asking permission]

JAN: *Not really.*

JENNY: ***Would you like*** *some time, and we can come back to you?* [asking permission]

JAN: *No, it's fine. Let's hear it.*

ALEXANDRA: *I thought it was great! The client seemed happy and really liked you!*

JENNY: *Jan did do a good job. Alexandra,* ***could you provide*** *a specific empathy example for Jan?* [asking permission]

ALEXANDRA: *Sure, after the client said something about being up all night with her baby, you said, "You must be **exhausted**."*

JENNY: *That's a great example. Alexandra, **what** would you do in a situation like this?* [open-ended inquiry]

ALEXANDRA: As soon as I walk into the room and see a baby carrier, I introduce myself to the client, offer congratulations, and ask, *"Tell me about the new addition to your family."*

JENNY: *Alexandra, **Let's take a minute** to role-play that, to see how it goes.* [signpost] *Jan, **would you** step into the role of the client?* [asking permission] *Let's give it a **try**.* [signpost] ***How** did that go for you, Alexandra < debrief role-play>?* [open-ended inquiry]

Now, let's hear from Nigel. [signpost]

NIGEL: *You should have offered to bring in an assistant with toys to help entertain the baby up front.*

JAN: *What assistant? What toys? When would I have the time to do all that?*

JENNY: ***Let's back up** a minute.* [signpost] *Nigel, **may I** share an observation on your feedback?* [asking permission]

NIGEL: *Sure.*

JENNY: ***I heard** your feedback start with "You should have. . .,"* [reflective listening] *which can put people on the defensive. **I'm wondering** if you might reword it as a suggestion rather than a directive.* [asking permission]

NIGEL: *Ah, I could say, I noticed the client's baby was distracting for you and the client. If I can offer a suggestion?* [Pause] *It might've been supportive to offer the client help maybe offer to bring in an assistant with toys to help entertain the baby. Does that work?*

JENNY: *That's it exactly! And Nigel, **what** was your favorite open-ended inquiry?* [open-ended inquiry]

NIGEL: *I thought it was perceptive when Jan asked, "Tell me how Beau is doing with the new baby in the household." We learned that Beau is anxious and skittish around the baby. It provided an opportunity for Jan to help with Beau's acclimation.*

Talk Through Technology – Video Recording

Video recording is the communication coach's technology of choice, as self-perception lacks accuracy. We learn a lot from watching a video recording of our own and others' performances. Reviewing video recordings allows us to see ourselves more clearly; provides a chance for specific, descriptive coaching and feedback in the moment; and demonstrates skills for others. A full description of how to set up and conduct communication rounds or a video review session is provided in Chapter 11.

The hidden gift of video review is the "eye spy" or "fly-on-the-wall" observation point. From this objective angle, we spot examples of effective verbal communication, identify missed opportunities to use skills, and assess nonverbal communication behaviors. We notice distracting nonverbal gestures, lengths of pauses, interruptions, and excessive use of minimal encouragers or filler words (e.g. *okay, um, uh, like, absolutely, great, awesome*). Watching video recordings over time enables us to track communication skill development and our progress implementing new skills or approaches.

Today, video recording technology – Go-Pros, iPads, smartphones, tablets, and video surveillance technology – is affordable, accessible, unobtrusive, mobile, and convenient. We provide recommendations below for how to video record client interactions in the examination room (Box 9.11).

Box 9.11   Tips for Video Recording in the Examination Room

---

1. Obtain oral or written, client or colleague **consent** prior to video recording. If you are video recording on a regular basis, we advise obtaining legal advice from practice counsel to create a formal client- or colleague-consent process and form. Include the following key pieces of information:

   a. Purpose of the video recording, including benefits to patients, clients, and the veterinary team.
   I am improving my communication skills, and it would be helpful to review a video recording of today's appointment. The purpose is to identify my communication strengths and areas for growth so I can serve clients and patients of the practice better.

   b. How the video recording will be used, and who will view it.
   I will review the video with my communication coach or with a small group of colleagues, who'll provide feedback on my communication with you.

   c. Where the video recording will be stored, and for how long.
   The video will be stored for two weeks on a secure, password-protected computer until our video-review meeting is completed.

   d. Assurance that the video recording will be deleted post-exercise.
   After the meeting, I will delete the video from our computer files, and no copies will be made, distributed, or used elsewhere.

   e. Confirmation that the video recording will be kept confidential and used only for training purposes.
   The video will not be shared with anyone else and will be used only for my communication development.

   f. Assurance for the client that the video recording will not interfere with the client service or patient care received.
   The videorecording will not distract me or interfere with the flow of our appointment; you and (pet's name) will receive the same great care you always do.

   g. Request for client or colleague consent.
   Would it be all right with you if I video record today's appointment?

2. Consider the **placement** of the video camera in the examination or meeting room to capture nonverbal communication. For coaching purposes, we are most interested in observing the nonverbal behaviors of the veterinary professional working on their communication skills over those of the client or colleague. Therefore, place the camera so it is facing the veterinary professional, to allow for assessment of eye contact, facial expressions, gestures, body language, distance, and positioning. Use a tripod or mounting bracket to get the right position, angle, and height of the video camera.

3. Account for the distance between the video camera and the speaker to preserve **audio quality**. Conduct a pilot test to ensure that the microphone clearly receives the voices over the veterinary practice background noise. Achieving high-quality audio is instrumental in recording the verbal communication skills used or the client cue missed.

4. **Position** the video equipment to ensure camera safety. Curious patients may jump onto the examination room counter and bump the tripod and video camera or knock them onto the floor.

5. Save **video recordings** temporarily on a secure, password-protected computer for the time between capture and video review. After the video-review session, delete the video recording from the computer, including emptying it from the computer's trash bin. It is a privacy violation to make or share copies of the videos.

Put the Coaching Skills into Practice

In this chapter, we revisit the communication styles exercises from Chapter 2. The focus in Chapter 2 was on client and colleague communication styles in client and veterinary professional interactions. In this chapter, we hone in on colleague relations and repeat communication styles, this time in the setting of intra-professional communication coaching. This is a purposefully built-in redundancy to apply key lessons of communication styles to coaching, feedback, and workplace dynamics.

Do-It-Yourself Exercises

For the following exercises, refer to Figure 2.1 in Chapter 2.

Exercise 9.1 Skill Spot-Communication Styles

Following are quotes from various colleagues. Identify which of the two communication styles, expert or partner, is reflected in each quote. The answer key is at the end of the chapter.

1. *I'd like to work with you on enhancing time management. What ideas do you have to start?*

2. *What you should do is . . .*

3. *You ought to introduce yourself to every client.*

4. *I am sensing your stress right now. Would you like to take a break and come back in a few minutes?*

5. *What would you like to try?*

6. *We need to start with getting the client's agenda up front.*

Exercise 9.2 Self-Assessment

1. Reflect on recent coaching interactions with one or more of the colleagues on your immediate team that you would like to explore in depth. Identify an example of when the interaction was on track and when it went off the rails.

2. For each example, follow these steps:
   a. What was your communication style?
   b. What one word would you use to characterize the interaction (e.g. awkward, tense, relaxed, or mutual)?
   c. What verbal and nonverbal cues indicated that the interaction was (awkward, tense, relaxed, or mutual)?
   d. How did it align with the partner communication style used in coaching?
   e. How might you adjust your approach next time to align even more with the partner communication coaching style?

f. What specifically would you repeat or would you do differently in your next interaction to support being a successful coach? List three concrete verbal or nonverbal behaviors, and create example phrases for each verbal behavior so they are at the ready.

Engage-the-Entire-Team Exercise

Exercise 9.3   Reflect, Share, and Discuss Your Preferred Coaching Experience

1. Gather your immediate team or the entire practice team together.

2. Ask everyone to self-reflect and identify a time when they were coached effectively:
   a. During this coaching interaction:
      i. How was feedback provided?
      ii. What is one thing that contributed to an effective coaching and feedback session?
      iii. What is one thing that did not contribute to an effective coaching and feedback session, if any?

3. Ask each person to briefly present their experience and thoughts to the group so the entire team hears what contributes to enhanced coaching and feedback.

4. Next, ask each person to share one thing that is working well and one opportunity for growth in relation to their current approach to coaching and feedback.

5. Close this exercise with time to reflect and then share individual commitments out loud:
   a. What will you do to meet the coaching needs of your colleagues?
   b. When someone's approach to coaching or feedback is not in alignment for you, how will you ask for something different?

6. Create a follow-up plan for moving forward. How will you track progress, recognize accomplishments, and set objectives for next steps?

Take It Away

1. Be aware of, and knowledgeable about, your **coaching approach** and how it aligns with the partner communication style. Be flexible, stretch, and adapt when necessary.
2. Ensure **feedback is specific, descriptive, balanced, and relevant** to colleagues' communication objectives.
3. Be **receptive to feedback**; ask for clarification, specific examples, and other viewpoints when necessary.
4. Stick closely to the **coaching process**; these proven steps guide the coach role and provide a clear, consistent, and predictable approach to put colleagues at ease.
5. Empower colleagues, **elicit colleague's perspective,** and invite them to collaborate, brainstorm, problem-solve, and propose solutions.

Answer Key

Exercise 9.1   Skill Spot-Communication Styles

1. *I'd like to work with you on enhancing time management. What ideas do you have to start?* [partner]

2. *What you should do is . . .*[expert]

3. *You ought to introduce yourself to every client.* [expert]

4. *I am sensing your stress right now. Would you like to take a break and come back in a few minutes?* [partner]

5. *What would you like to try?* [partner]

6. *We need to start with getting the client's agenda up front.* [expert]

References

Adams, C.L. and Kurtz, S. (2012). Coaching, and feedback: Enhancing communication teaching and learning in veterinary practice settings. *J. Vet. Med. Educ.* 39 (3): 217–228. https://doi.org/10.3138/jvme.0512-038R.

Barbour, A. (2000). *Making Contact or Making Sense: Functional and Dysfunctional Ways of Relating*. Humanities Institute Lecture 1999–2000 Series. Colorado: University of Denver.

Brookhart, S.M. (2017). *How to Give Effective Feedback to Your Students*, 2ed. Alexandria, VA: ASCD.

Cornell, K.K., Coe, J.B., Shaw, D.H. et al. (2019). Investigation of the effects of a practice-level communication program on veterinary health-care team members' communication confidence, client satisfaction, and practice financial metrics. *J. Am. Vet. Med. Assoc.* 255 (12): 1377–1388. https://doi.org/10.2460/javma.255.12.1377.

Covey, S.R. (2004). *The 7 Habits of Highly Effective People: Restoring Character Ethic*. New York, NY: Free Press.

Dweck, C. (2016). *Mindset: The New Psychology of Success. How We Can Learn to Fulfill Our Potential*. New York, NY: Random House.

Hunter L.J. and Shaw J.R.S. (2016). Role-Playing: Learn skils by acting out. *Veterinary Team Brief*. July. 49–52.

Hunter, L.J. and Shaw, J.R.S. (2018a). Feedback: The art is in the delivery. *Veterinary Team Brief*. October: 33–36.

Hunter, L.J. and Shaw, J.R.S. (2018b). The art of receiving feedback. *Veterinary Team Brief*. November/December: 14–16.

Janke, N., Shaw, J.R., and Coe, J.B. (2022). On-site communication skills education increases appointment-specific client satisfaction in four companion animal practices in Texas. *J. Am. Vet. Med. Assoc.* 260 (13): 1711–1720. https://doi.org/10.2460/javma.22.06.0242.

Janke, N., Shaw, J.R., and Coe, J.B. (2023). On-site communication skills education increases client-centered communication in four companion animal practices. *J. Am. Vet. Med. Assoc.* 261 (9): 1–11. https://doi.org/10.2460/javma.23.02.0101.

Kinnison, T., May, S.A., and Guile, D. (2014). Inter-professional practice: From veterinarian to the veterinary team. *J. Vet. Med. Educ.* 41 (2): 172–178. https://doi.org/10.3138/jvme.0713-095R2.

Kurtz, S., Silverman, J., and Draper, J. (2005). *Teaching and Learning Communication Skills in Medicine*. London, England: CRC Press.

Moore, I.C., Coe, J.B., Adams, C.L. et al. (2014). The role of veterinary team effectiveness in job satisfaction and burnout in companion animal veterinary clinics. *J. Am. Vet. Med. Assoc.* 245 (5): 513–524. https://doi.org/10.2460/javma.245.5.513.

Pizzolon, C.N., Coe, J.B., and Shaw, J.S. (2019). Evaluation of team effectiveness and personal empathy for associations with professional quality of life and job satisfaction in companion animal practice personnel. *J. Am. Vet. Med. Assoc.* 254 (10): 1204–1217. https://doi.org/10.2460/javma.254.10.1204.

Shaw, J.R., Barley, G.E., Broadfoot, K. et al. (2016). Outcome assessment of onsite communication skills education in a companion animal practice. *J. Am. Vet. Med. Assoc.* 249 (4): 419–432. https://doi.org/10.2460/javma.249.4.419.

Shaw, J.R., Barley, G.E., Hill, A.E. et al. (2010). Communication skills education onsite in a veterinary practice. *Patient Educ. Couns.* 80 (3): 337–344. https://doi.org/10.1016/j.pec.2010.06.012.

Stone, D. and Heen, S. (2014). *Thanks for the Feedback: The Science and Art of Receiving Feedback Well*. New York, NY: Penguin Group.

10

Transferring the Skills to Various Contexts

Abstract

The advantage of taking a skills-based approach to communication training and development is that it provides an assorted toolbox to be carried into every conversation, albeit routine or challenging or with a client or colleague. With competence, the veterinary professional assesses the scenario, grabs the appropriate communication tool(s), puts them into practice, and reflects afterward on what worked. With a sturdy and agile toolbox, the skills are ready for various circumstances and transferable to all client and colleague conversations. In the previous chapters, we outlined a myriad of routine and challenging client and team conversations. Here we select a handful of crucial conversations with clients and colleagues and provide further examples of the communication tools in action for each specific context.

Introduction

The advantage of taking a skills-based approach to communication training and development is that it provides an assorted toolbox of communication skills to be carried into every conversation, albeit routine or challenging or with a client or colleague. With competence, the veterinary professional assesses the scenario, grabs the appropriate communication tool(s), puts them into practice, and reflects afterward on what worked. With a sturdy and agile toolbox, the skills are ready for various circumstances and transferable to all client and colleague conversations.

In the previous chapters, we outlined a myriad of routine and challenging client and team conversations. Here we select a handful of crucial conversations and provide further examples of the communication tools in action with clients and colleagues. The intent is to illustrate how the communication skills might be used in these situations. Having developed the core communication skills presented in this book, we prepare and equip you to tackle these and any other difficult conversations.

A crucial conversation involves volatile emotions, opposing opinions, or high stakes (Patterson et al. 2012). All of these factors are in place when an animal's health is at risk, the client and veterinary team do not see eye to eye, or the human–animal bond is fragile. The same is true for veterinary professional interactions, when appointments are overbooked, the team is short-staffed, or conflict goes unmanaged. When emotions run high, the interaction quickly escalates. Be mindful

Developing Communication Skills for Veterinary Practice, First Edition. Jane R. Shaw and Jason B. Coe.
© 2024 John Wiley & Sons, Inc. Published 2024 by John Wiley & Sons, Inc.

of throwing gas on the fire. Purposefully and carefully choose communication skills to diffuse emotion, partner with the other person, and support a stepwise approach.

Scenarios

This chapter highlights six **client conversations**:

1. Tackle tough topics
2. Support grief and address anger
3. Deliver bad news
4. Facilitate euthanasia discussions
5. Disclose medical errors
6. Discuss finances

We also present six **team conversations**:

1. Promote inclusivity
2. Elicit colleague's perspective
3. Set boundaries
4. Motivate colleagues
5. Create a toxic-free practice
6. Address workplace bullying

In each of these crucial conversations, many of the same communication skills are used, just in a different context. The scenarios exemplify the utility of the communication skills introduced throughout this book and emphasize the importance of honing each tool. We outline essential steps to these difficult conversations, recognizing that they are not linear as laid out here. Rather, we need to constantly evaluate the direction of the conversation, assess our client's or colleague's response, and remain flexible in our approach. Skillfully manage these challenging topics to engender confidence, demonstrate compassion, foster connection, build trust, and enhance professional fulfillment and well-being.

Client Conversations

Tackle Tough Topics

Set the Scene: Muffuletta, a 6-month-old, female terrier mix, and her caregiver, Shawna, arrive for a pre-surgical appointment for her ovariohysterectomy. During the weight check, Muffuletta growls and snaps at the veterinary technician. This is her "second offense," as she showed aggression when she was in the clinic for final puppy vaccinations. Shawna immediately begins to cry (Hunter and Shaw 2014a).

Some topics are tough because they involve discussing subjects that clients may perceive as a reflection of their care for their pet or that may be directly related to client actions that are contributing to the problem. Weight management, parasites, dental hygiene, and behavior are a few of these sensitive topics. Avoid finger-pointing, and instead elicit the client's point of view and offer partnership to develop a plan together. Place yourself in the client's shoes, and ask open-ended inquiries to understand their thoughts, opinions, concerns, and values surrounding the topic to be addressed (Sidebars 10.1 and 10.2).

Sidebar 10.1   Communication Skills to Tackle Tough Topics

Empathy

Reflective listening

Open-ended inquiry

Partnership

Signpost

Asking permission

Chunk-and-check

End summary

Contracts for next steps

Final check

Sidebar 10.2   Essential Steps to Tackle Tough Topics

Given the potential for judgment in this conversation, it is important to empathize, proceed with caution, and understand where the client is coming from.

1. Establish initial rapport.
2. Elicit the client's perspective.
3. Empathize, partner, and support the client.
4. Share your concerns, and ask permission to discuss.
5. Seek common ground, offer alternatives, and engage in shared decision-making.
6. Summarize and strategize.

1. **Establish initial rapport.**
   I see how worked you are about Muffuletta's behavior. [empathy]
   You've been working hard with Muffuletta. [reflective listening]
   I can only imagine your disappointment when something like this happens; it feels like a setback. [empathy]

2. **Elicit the client's perspective.**
   What are your thoughts about Muffuletta's behavior? [open-ended inquiry]
   How are you dealing with Muffuletta's behavior? [open-ended inquiry]
   What is working for you and Muffuletta? [open-ended inquiry]
   What have you learned about Muffuletta's behavior? [open-ended inquiry]

3. **Empathize, partner, and support the client.**
   I see that you are upset, and I know this is a difficult topic. [empathy]
   We will work together to address Muffuletta's behavior. [partnership]
   It sounds like Muffuletta wants to learn and please you. [reflective listening]

4. **Share your concerns, and ask permission to discuss.**
   Shawna, I am also concerned about what just happened with Muffuletta. [signpost]
   Can we talk more about it? [asking permission]
   This is the second time I am aware of that Muffuletta showed aggression toward clinic staff, and I'm worried it is not improving. [chunk] *What other incidents are you aware of?* [check]

5. **Seek common ground, offer alternatives, and engage in shared decision-making.**

   *I have a few resources I'd like to share as a starting point **if you are open to it**.* [asking permission]

6. **Summarize and strategize.**

   You shared with me *that Muffuletta is your first pet, and you are concerned about her increasingly aggressive behavior, which worsened since you started traveling. You've tried some strategies that don't seem to be working and you're seeking urgent support.* [end summary]

   Our plan is to *enroll Muffuletta in a boarding facility with doggie daycare and training classes onsite. You'll attend obedience classes together when you are not on the road. And they will work with Muffuletta when you are on the road and she's boarding. I will provide you with a list of boarding facilities with trainers to interview.* [contracts for next steps]

   How *does that sound to you?* [final check]

Support Grief and Address Anger

Set the Scene: A deep red color is creeping up Mr. Russo's neck. Sergeant, his four-year-old male-castrated mastiff, was diagnosed with gastric dilatation and volvulus. Mr. Russo points a shaking finger between your eyes as he says loudly, *No! You must do more! You can't just let him die!* (Hunter and Shaw 2015a).

Clients angry with grief are sometimes labeled "challenging." Keep in mind that they are in a challenging situation and are struggling to cope. Anger is a grief emotion that masks vulnerable feelings like sadness, helplessness, overwhelm, guilt or shame (Benson 2023). What appears tough on the outside is often hiding fear on the inside. It is important to recognize that these intense feelings are not directed at you, which is the first step to navigate difficult conversations. Expressing empathy through normalizing, validating, nonjudgmental statements, and employing appropriate self-disclosure can unmask the anger and reveal the underlying grief (Sidebars 10.3 and 10.4).

Sidebar 10.3   Communication Skills to Support Grief and Address Anger

Empathy

Partnership

Open-ended inquiry

Signpost

Chunk-and-check

Asking permission

Internal summary

End summary

Contracts for next steps

Final check

Sidebar 10.4   Essential Steps to Support Grief and Address Anger

Given the nature of this heated conversation, it is critical to diffuse emotion, establish trust, not take it personally, and move the interaction forward.

1. Acknowledge emotions, and establish initial rapport.
2. Elicit the client's knowledge and deliver information.
3. Share options.
4. Empathize, partner, and support the client.
5. Summarize and strategize.

1. **Acknowledge emotions, and establish initial rapport.**

    *I see you are **angry** and how much Sergeant **means to you,** and how **worried** you are about him.* [empathy]

    *We are working our hardest to prevent him from dying, and **I will make sure you are kept informed** all the way.* [partnership]

    *I'm glad that you brought Sergeant here when you did, so **we can support both of you**.* [partnership]

2. **Elicit the client's knowledge and deliver information.**

    ***What** do you know about bloat?* [open-ended inquiry]

    Sergeant is in critical condition. [signpost - warning shot]

    We are stabilizing him by giving fluids, addressing his pain, and relieving the pressure in his stomach. [chunk] ***What** questions can I address right now?* [check]

    *This **is a life-threatening disease** for Sergeant, **with the potential for complications**.* [signpost - warning shot]

    So, the faster we act, the better the chance that we can help him and achieve better outcomes. [chunk] ***What** additional information can I provide at this point?* [check]

3. **Share options.**

    ***Because time is of the essence** for Sergeant,* [signpost - warning shot] ***can we talk about** what we need to do to treat the bloat?* [asking permission]

    The option that can save Sergeant's life and resolve his bloat is surgery, and unfortunately, it's not a guarantee. [chunk] ***What** are your thoughts?* [check]

    ***The other option** is a difficult one.* [signpost - warning shot] *Euthanasia would ease Sergeant's suffering immediately and is an option **for us** to discuss at this time.* [partnership]

4. **Empathize, partner, and support the client.**

    *Euthanasia is a **heart-breaking** decision to consider.* [empathy]

    *You **responded quickly**, **brought Sergeant here**, and are **giving him the help** he needs now.* [internal summary]

    *I remember feeling so **angry** and **helpless** when my dog bloated.* [empathy]

    ***We will work closely with you** to do everything we can for Sergeant.* [partnership]

    ***Who** else can we call that you would like here to take part in the decision-making for Sergeant?* [open-ended inquiry]

5. **Summarize and strategize.**

    *After weighing the possible risks, **we decided to** take Sergeant to surgery.* [partnership] *And you would like to be kept posted on Sergeant's progress throughout the process.* [end summary]

    Before we prep him for surgery, you'll have a chance to visit with Sergeant briefly. Nina, my surgical assistant, will call you with an update once I've fully examined his stomach and nearby organs. Let me confirm that I have the correct contact information for you. [contracts for next steps]

    ***What** other concerns do you have before we go to surgery?* [final check]

Deliver Bad News

Set the Scene: Claire presents with Max, her beloved six-year-old, male-castrated yellow Labrador and hiking partner. Max is diagnosed with severe hip dysplasia. In the past, Claire shared numerous stories of their outdoor adventures and a long-anticipated trip to Alaska. Even though Max is otherwise healthy and happy, this new diagnosis will significantly change their lifestyle, activities, and future together (Allen and Shaw 2010).

Bad news is any information that negatively alters a person's views of their future (Buckman 1992). Clients' interpretations and responses to bad news are often tied to their relationship with their companion animal, past experiences, other life stressors, and support system. Some clients may react with anger or blame or overwhelming feelings of guilt, shock, disbelief, or sadness; others may appear calm, stoic, or under control. Keep in mind that bad news is in the mind of the beholder; what is bad news to one person is not necessarily bad news to another. Therefore, we approach the bad news conversation with presence, attention, and intention, and express empathy, offer partnership, and allow time for the client to process the information provided (Sidebars 10.5 and 10.6).

Sidebar 10.5   Communication Skills to Deliver Bad News

Preparation

Partnership

Empathy

Open-ended inquiry

Asking permission

Signpost

Chunk-and-check

End summary

Contracts for next steps

Final check

Sidebar 10.6   Essential Steps to Deliver Bad News

Given the sensitivity of this difficult conversation, it is paramount to keep it simple, go slow, seek your client's perspective often, offer partnership, and let the client set the pace.

1. Prepare.
2. Create a supportive setting.
3. Elicit the client's perspective.
4. Deliver the information.
5. Empathize, partner, and support the client.
6. Summarize and strategize.

1. **Prepare.** Take a breath to center and ground yourself to present a calm and focused demeanor and be fully present with your client and patient.

2. **Create a supportive setting.** Ensure privacy, minimize distractions, attend to client and patient comfort, establish rapport and trust, and gather client support.

> *I am glad that you brought Max in so* **we** *can address this problem* **together**. [partnership]
> **It sounds like** *that last hike was* **rough** *on both of you.* [empathy]
> **I am wondering** *who else may want to take part in this conversation.* [open-ended inquiry]

3. **Elicit the client's perspective.**

What concerns you most about Max? [open-ended inquiry]

What other information would be helpful to you at this time? [open-ended inquiry]

Claire, I know how involved you are in caring for Max. How much detail would you prefer I go into as we discuss his lameness? [open-ended inquiry]

How would you like to proceed? [open-ended inquiry]

4. **Deliver the information.**

Would it be all right to go over the X-ray findings with you? [asking permission]

Claire, what I saw on the X-rays is concerning. [signpost - warning shot]

The X-rays show that Max has hip dysplasia, which is causing his lameness. That explains why he's had difficulty rising after his hikes. [chunk] *How does that fit with what you've been thinking?* [check]

5. **Empathize, partner, and support the client.**

I can imagine how hard this is to hear. Max has been such a good hiking buddy. [empathy]

This must come as quite a shock, given how active you both are. [empathy]

I'm going to be with you and Max as we navigate these changes. [partnership]

6. **Summarize and strategize.**

Unfortunately, today we diagnosed Max with hip dysplasia. The good news is that there are multiple effective management options. Your goals are to address Max's pain, strengthen his hind-end muscles, and get him back on the trail. [end summary]

We are going to start with a special diet, anti-inflammatory medications, joint supplements, and physical therapy. [contracts for next steps]

What other questions do you have about the plan for Max, before we move forward? [final check]

Facilitate Euthanasia Discussions

Set the Scene: The Ortegas brought in Manuel, their 12-year-old, male-castrated Old English Sheepdog in remission after treatment for lymphoma. They felt his lymph nodes again and are concerned that the cancer is back. And worse, Manuel is refusing to eat, is not interested in going out for walks, and spends most of the day sleeping. They are wondering if it is time to euthanize Manuel (Shaw et al. 2009/2010).

The term euthanasia is derived from the Greek words *eu*, which means "good," and *thanatos*, meaning "death." (Lagoni et al. 1994) Euthanasia is a humane, painless gift of peace for a beloved pet. End-of-life discussions clarify the client's wishes, minimize regrets, foster decision-making, and allow the client to cope better with the death of their pet. (Matte et al. 2020). Veterinary professionals are emotionally impacted as well by a pet's illness or impending death. How end-of-life conversations are conducted strengthens our relationship with our clients, enhances clients' ability to manage (Matte et al. 2019) and promotes professional wellness. This conversation entails support, collaboration, slow delivery, time to process, and regularly checking in with the client (Sidebars 10.7 and 10.8).

Sidebar 10.7   Communication Skills to Facilitate Euthanasia Discussions

Reflective listening

Empathy

Open-ended inquiry

Asking permission

Chunk-and-check

Signpost

Partnership

End summary

Contracts for next steps

Final check

Sidebar 10.8   Essential Steps to Facilitate a Euthanasia Discussion

Given the fragility of euthanasia discussions, it is crucial to proceed slowly and with sensitivity, discuss decisions step by step, and empathize, partner, and support the client.

1. Establish initial rapport.
2. Elicit the client's perspective.
3. Share your patient assessment.
4. Present the euthanasia option.
5. Empathize, partner, and support the client.
6. Explain the euthanasia process and related decisions.
7. Summarize and strategize.

1. **Establish initial rapport.**

   *You have taken such **good care** of Manuel throughout his cancer.* [reflective listening]
   *__I see__ how much you **love** him.* [empathy]

2. **Elicit the client's perspective.**

   ***How** do you feel Manuel is doing?* [open-ended inquiry]
   ***What** are the other members of your household thinking?* [open-ended inquiry]

3. **Share your patient assessment.**

   ***Would you like** me to share what I'm seeing, as I haven't seen Manuel for three weeks?* [asking permission]
   He has lost more weight, seems less responsive and more uncomfortable. [chunk] ***What** are your impressions of him?* [check]
   *While I can give him more medication for his pain, **unfortunately,** his body is declining due to the cancer.* [signpost - warning shot]

4. **Present the euthanasia option.**

   ***You brought up** the question of euthanasia earlier.* [reflective listening]
   *Euthanasia is one of the **most difficult decisions** we face in caring for our pets.* [signpost - warning shot]
   ***I am wondering whether** it would be all right with you if we took a few minutes to discuss euthanasia.* [asking permission]
   ***What** previous experiences have you had with euthanasia?* [open-ended inquiry]

5. **Empathize, partner, and support the client.**

> *Making a euthanasia decision on Manuel's behalf is **challenging**. It can feel **overwhelming** to determine what's best for Manuel and your family.* [empathy]
>
> *I **will be here** to support you and Manuel.* [partnership]
>
> *I **fully support** your decision and will honor your wishes for Manuel.* [partnership]
>
> *It **is hard to imagine** life without Manuel. I can see how **close** you are to him.* [empathy]

6. **Explain the euthanasia process and related decisions** (Box 10.1).

> *I **am wondering if** it would be all right with you if I were to walk you through the euthanasia process we use at our clinic.* [asking permission]
>
> *I would like to ensure that we **prepare ahead of time** by going over everything that will happen during his euthanasia.* [signpost]
>
> *There are **several decisions** to make in relation to the euthanasia procedure.* [signpost]
>
> *I **am wondering if** you'd like to talk about them now.* [asking permission]

Box 10.1 Euthanasia-Related Decisions to Consider

__Who__ would like to be present during the euthanasia? [open-ended inquiry]
__Where__ would you like the euthanasia procedure to take place? [closed-ended inquiry]
__Who__ would you like to conduct the euthanasia procedure? [closed-ended inquiry]
__What__ spiritual observances would you like to include? [open-ended inquiry]
__Would you like to__ consider a necropsy to determine the cause of death? [asking permission]
__What__ are your plans to care for Manuel's body? [open-ended inquiry]
__Would you like__ a clay paw print or hair clipping? [asking permission]
__How__ would you like to memorialize Manuel? [open-ended inquiry]

---

7. **Summarize and strategize.**

> *Let me reflect on what I heard. You would like to be outside in the garden with Manuel on his bed with his favorite blanket and toy. You have a special poem the children would like to read. You'd like us to make a paw print, and you plan to plant Manuel's ashes under a tree.* [end summary]
>
> *Today is not the day to say goodbye to Manuel. I've provided you with additional pain medication, clinic hours, and an at-home euthanasia service in case of emergency. You will call to schedule the appointment once your family has had more time with Manuel.* [contracts for next steps]
>
> *How else can I support you, your family, and Manuel?* [final check]

Disclose Medical Errors

Set the Scene: After struggling to retrieve the ovaries during the first cat spay of the day, Dr. Jackson requests gender identification of Sophie, a young tabby cat. Molly, the technician reads the collar under the drape, frowns, apologizes, and shares that the patient is Sam, a male neutered tabby cat, with feline asthma that was in the hospital for a thoracic radiograph (Allen and Shaw 2011).

A medical error is a mistake that results in a breach to the standard of care for a patient. When this happens, we breathe, center ourselves, and calm our initial reaction. As appropriate, we advise employers, professional liability insurance, and legal counsel and consult our colleagues for support. Then we take the first step to address the client; pick up the phone or invite the client to a private setting, such as an examination room or office. We approach this conversation with humility and honesty, and draw on the use of empathy, partnership, and chunk-and-check from our toolbox (Sidebars 10.9 and 10.10).

Sidebar 10.9   Key Communication Skills to Disclose Medical Errors

Signpost

Asking permission

Empathy

Chunk-and-check

Partnership

End summary

Contracts for next steps

Final check

Sidebar 10.10   Essential Steps to Disclose Medical Errors

Given the pressure of this difficult conversation, it is urgent to apologize early, empathize often, check in with the client repeatedly, and follow the client's lead.

1. Provide a warning shot.
2. Disclose all information about the error, including what happened and why it happened.
3. Take responsibility for the error.
4. Apologize, empathize, and express remorse.
5. Explain the implications of the error for the patient.
6. Address how future errors will be prevented, and make restitution.

---

1. **Provide a warning shot.**

   Mr. Singh, **I need to speak with you** *about Sam.* [signpost - warning shot] *First, I want to assure you that Sam is okay.* **Is now a good time**? [asking permission]

2. **Disclose all information about the error, including what happened and why it happened.**

   I'm going to share some news with you that is likely to be **distressing**. [signpost - warning shot] *You brought Sam in today for chest X-rays to assess his asthma. Unfortunately, I mistook him for a female tabby kitty who was in our hospital to be spayed and I mistakenly tried to spay Sam.* [chunk] **This comes as** *quite a* **shock**. [empathy] **What** *questions do you have?* [check] *It was at the beginning of the surgical procedure, once I entered his abdomen, that I realized my mistake.* **Shall I continue?** [asking permission]

3. **Take responsibility for the error.**

   You probably are asking yourself, "How could this happen?" and **I will explain further**. [signpost] *It was my fault that I did not double-check Sam's identification collar and gender before the procedure.* [chunk] **What** *else would you like to know?* [check]

4. **Apologize, empathize, and express remorse.**

   I am **so sorry** *that I made this mistake.*

*I hear your **disappointment** in me,* [empathy] *and I am also disappointed in myself.*
*I feel **terrible** that I have hurt Sam and our relationship.*

5. **Explain the implications of the error for the patient.**

    Sam has an abdominal incision that will require rest and monitoring. Most young cats recover well. I will dispense pain medication for discomfort, and he will need to wear a cone to protect the incision. [chunk] ***What** concerns do you have?* [check]

6. **Address how future errors will be prevented, and make restitution.**

    To prevent this from happening again, my colleagues and I created a new identification protocol to clarify the name and gender of all patients in our hospital. [chunk]. ***What** questions do you have about this?* [check]

    ***In summary**, I made a terrible surgical error that put Sam's health and your trust at risk. I will support Sam and yourself, in every way, throughout his recovery,* [partnership] *and I am grateful to you for allowing me to continue to care for Sam* [end summary]

    ***Going forward**, you will not pay for any expenses associated with the surgery, pain medication, cone, or recheck examination to monitor Sam's incision. At his recheck, If you are willing* [ask permission] *we will re-assess and can take chest X-rays to evaluate Sam's asthma* [contracts for next steps]

    ***What** else can I do to support you and Sam, and address my mistake?* [final check]

Discuss Finances

Set the Scene: Jengo is a 16-year-old, male-castrated Maine Coon cat with diabetes mellitus that progressed to ketoacidosis. The Charles family are dedicated and committed to Jengo's care, and the costs of the care are adding up (Hunter and Shaw 2018).

Financial discussions are uncomfortable from a veterinary professional and client perspective. For veterinary professionals, tension exists between providing necessary patient care, charging appropriately for services provided, and not being perceived to be all about the money. Clients prefer that the veterinary team focus on caring for their pet first, and the cost of the care second (Coe et al. 2007). The emotions associated with pet attachment, such as concern, fear, and guilt add further challenges to this conversation. Therefore, take time and care to build rapport through empathy and partnership before moving into this often-sensitive topic. Give clients time to consider the options by asking permission and using chunk-and-check, and determine which decisions are needed for immediate patient care and what can be resolved later (Sidebars 10.11 and 10.12).

Sidebar 10.11   Communication Skills to Discuss Finances

Signpost

Asking permission

Chunk-and-check

Partnership

Open-ended inquiry

Empathy

End summary

Contracts for next steps

Final check

Sidebar 10.12   Essential Steps to Discuss Finances

Given the personal nature of this difficult conversation, it is integral to present options, be flexible, identify alternatives, and collaborate with the client.

1. Provide treatment options.
2. Present a written care plan or value matrix, including the associated costs.
3. Highlight the value – the impact on the patient's health and well-being.
4. Make a recommendation.
5. Discuss the alternatives and support shared decision-making.
6. Elicit the client's perspective.
7. Empathize, partner, and support the client.
8. Summarize and strategize.

1. **Provide treatment options.**

   Let's go through *the treatment options, advantages and disadvantages, and associated costs together.* [signpost]

2. **Present a written care plan or value matrix, including the associated costs.**

   Would you like to *go over the care plan together?* [asking permission]

   I've put it into a chart format *based on each option, the advantages and disadvantages and the costs, to make it easier for us to visualize everything at once.* [signpost]

3. **Highlight the value – the impact on the patient's health and well-being.**

   I would like to *share my thoughts behind each option and how they will impact Jengo's quality of life.* [signpost].

4. **Make a recommendation.**

   My recommendation is to hospitalize Jengo, perform bloodwork, administer anti-nausea medication, and start fluid therapy, so we can help Jengo feel better. [chunk] ***How*** *does that sound to you?* [check]

5. **Discuss the alternatives, and support shared decision-making.**

   If you are not sure about hospitalization, ***would it be helpful to*** *further discuss some of the other options we could consider for Jengo's care?* [asking permission]

6. **Elicit the client's perspective.**

   Before [signpost] ***we*** [partnership] *make any decisions,* ***I wonder if we*** [partnership] *could discuss your financial expectations for Jengo's care.* [asking permission]

   How *might this option fit into your family's budget?* [open-ended inquiry]

7. **Empathize, partner, and support the client.**

   I hear *that you are feeling financially* ***stretched*** *given all that you've done for Jengo.* [empathy]

   I wish too *that Jengo was not so sick.* [empathy]

   Balancing the care you want for Jengo against finances can be ***difficult.*** [empathy]

   We *will* ***work together*** *on a plan that provides the support Jengo needs and fits into your budget.* [partnership]

8. **Summarize and strategize.**

> ***From what you shared*** *and my physical examination, Jengo's diabetes has progressed. Fluids will rehydrate him, and anti-nausea medications will help Jengo feel better and hopefully get him eating again. At this time, you are concerned about the costs associated with hospitalization.* [end summary]
>
> ***You've elected to*** *hospitalize Jengo and treat him for the next 24 hours to see how he responds. I will call with a progress report tomorrow morning, and we can determine where to go from there, pending how Jengo is doing. I realize that this has been a stressful visit and this was a difficult decision to come to.* [empathy] [contracts for next steps]
>
> ***What*** *remaining questions do you have?* [final check]

Team Conversations

Promote Inclusivity

Set the Scene: Chris is a veterinary technician who is a recent addition and asset to the practice. At a recent staff meeting, Chris shared their personal pronouns with the rest of the veterinary team as they/them. Since then, Chris overheard several staff reference them in conversation as "she" or "her." Chris raises their experience with the practice manager.

Diversity is defined as differences between people, including, but not limited to: national origin, language, race, color, disability, ethnicity, age, religion, sexual orientation, gender identity, socioeconomic status, veteran status, and family structures (Denboba, 1993). Based on these differences, equity and inclusion involve developing the knowledge, skills, and behaviors to examine and consider our own biases, privileges, assumptions, and values, while seeking to examine and learn about systemic oppression, both historically and contemporarily. This continued commitment to equity-mindedness (Bensimon et al. 2016) allows us to foster inclusion. Inclusive team members practice self-discovery; seek continued education related to diversity, equity, and inclusion; promote allyship; and embrace necessary conversations with open, honest communication that involves asking permission, empathy, open-ended inquiry, and reflective listening (Sidebars 10.13 and 10.14) (Hunter and Shaw 2016).

Sidebar 10.13   Communication Skills to Be Inclusive

Empathy

Partnership

Asking permission

End Summary

Contracts for next steps

Final check

Sidebar 10.14   Essential Steps to Be Inclusive

To promote inclusivity; create a judgment-free zone that conveys support and demonstrates being an advocate.

1. Acknowledge your colleague's trust and experience.
2. Empathize, partner, and support your colleague.
3. Educate yourself and your team.
4. Summarize and strategize.

1. **Acknowledge your colleague's trust and experience**

   Thank you for trusting me enough to share this with me. ***It's disappointing*** *that we have not created an inclusive environment.* [empathy]

2. **Empathize, partner, and support your colleague.**

   I am hearing that you're not feeling ***welcomed*** *and* ***accepted*** *by the team* [empathy].
   You are a valuable member of this ***team,*** *and* ***I am committed to you*** *and to making this an inclusive environment.* [partnership]

3. **Educate yourself and your team.**

   Would you feel comfortable if *we invited an expert in to talk about the importance of using correct pronouns with our team?* [asking permission]

4. **Summarize and strategize.**

   From our conversation*, I am going to work to create an inclusive work environment. Unfortunately, it does not feel like a safe workplace for you, and I'm grateful to you for bringing your experience to my attention and allowing me the opportunity to address this with the team.* [end summary]
   For next steps*, I personally will take responsibility for fostering a more inclusive work environment, and I will address this with the team at our next team meeting. As part of this, I will also arrange diversity, equity, and inclusion training opportunities for the entire team within the next month.* [contracts for next steps]
   How *else can I support you?* [final check]

Elicit Colleague's Perspective

Set the Scene: Dr. Shima Quan, the practice owner, arrives early, works through the day with her head down, rarely takes lunch, and stays late unfaltering day after day. On the other hand, the new associate, Dr. Brad Harrison, is seeking a more balanced lifestyle, working a 32-hour week with three-day weekends and regular vacations (Shaw and Hunter 2015a).

At times, colleagues may be separated by different perspectives – attitudes, ethics, values, and paradigms. Yet, they share the same mission – a dedication to the health and well-being of colleagues, patients, and clients – which ultimately brings the two together. We build a bridge with our colleagues through patience, curiosity, and partnership (Sidebars 10.15 and 10.16).

Sidebar 10.15   Communication Skills to Elicit Colleague's Perspective

Open-ended inquiry

Asking permission

Empathy

Partnership

Chunk-and-check

End summary

Contracts for next steps

Final check

Sidebar 10.16   Essential Steps to Elicit Colleague's Perspective

To elicit colleague's perspective: seek common ground, to understand where our colleagues are coming from, and empathize and partner to seek a mutual solution moving forward.

1. Seek out your colleague's perspective.
2. Ask permission to discuss.
3. Empathize, partner, and support your colleague.
4. Share your concerns.
5. Summarize and strategize.

1. **Seek out your colleague's perspective.**
   How are things going since you joined our practice? [open-ended inquiry]
   *I would like to **hear more about** your career goals and aspirations* <ask about one at a time>. [open-ended inquiry]
   ***What** brings you the greatest fulfillment at work?* [open-ended inquiry]
   ***Share with me** how I can work with you to ease your concerns.* [open-ended inquiry]

2. **Ask permission to discuss.**
   ***Can we talk about** what we expect from each other as colleagues and from the practice?* <ask one at a time> [asking permission]
   ***I am wondering** if we can discuss your thoughts on how we can balance scheduling.* [asking permission]

3. **Empathize, partner, and support your colleague.**
   *I sense that working late is **difficult** for you and your family.* [empathy]
   *I understand that your **job is only one facet** of your life.* [empathy]
   *I could **learn a lot from you** about self-care.* [partnership]

4. **Share your concerns.**
   I can see we are both experiencing exhaustion and frustration in meeting the growing caseload and demanding schedule. [chunk] ***How** can we care for the team, clients, and patients, as well as our own professional wellness?* [check]
   I am concerned one or the other of us is here early and late day after day. We are missing important time with our families. [chunk] ***How** can we adjust the schedule so that it serves both our needs?* [check]

5. **Summarize and strategize.**
   ***It sounds like** we are both feeling stretched to balance our workload. We've both been working long days. We identified a relief valve in that mornings are more flexible for you and evenings more so for me.* [end summary]
   ***Going ahead**, it sounds like you're willing to start early to examine hospitalized patients, check-in surgical cases, and see emergencies before scheduled appointments. I will stay late in the evenings to conduct treatments for hospitalized patients, discharge surgery patients, and see emergencies until closing.* [contracts for next steps]
   ***How** do you think that will work?* [final check]

Set Boundaries

Set the Scene: This is the fourth client and patient in three weeks that required care well into the evening hours. Bianca, a devout veterinary technician, missed homework, dinner, and bedtime again with her partner and children. The once-complimentary nickname "client whisperer" is no longer received with a smile (Shaw and Hunter 2015b). In the following scenario, Bianca sets boundaries with a client (Mrs. Sangweni and Peaches), a colleague (Karina), and the practice owner (Dr. Macaluso).

Boundaries are the physical, emotional, social, and cognitive limits that separate one individual from another (Ashforth et al. 2000). Boundaries draw a line between where we end and another person begins to navigate healthy relationships. Maintaining strong boundaries creates constructive work environments by setting standards for behavior and reduces regret and resentment that result from boundary crossings (Sidebars 10.17 and 10.18).

The three main types of workplace boundaries are: (Criminal Watch Dog 2023)

1. **Job responsibilities:** Defined tasks in the job description
2. **Interpersonal boundaries:** Guided interactions with colleagues in the workplace
3. **Personal boundaries:** Protected time with family, friends, hobbies, and self-care outside of work

Sidebar 10.17   Communication Skills to Set Boundaries

Partnership
Empathy
Open-ended inquiry
End summary
Contracts for next steps
Final check

Sidebar 10.18   Essential Steps to Set Boundaries

To set boundaries: clearly state what you can do and need, seek your client's or colleague's perspective, and partner in establishing boundaries.

1. Use "I" statements to set limits and state what you can do.
2. Empathize, partner, and support your client or colleague.
3. Seek your client's or colleague's perspective.
4. Summarize and strategize.

1. **Use "I" statements to set limits and state what you can do.**
    *Mrs. Sangweni, **unfortunately I cannot be present** at Peaches' appointment. Before I leave, **I will provide you** with information on a cancer support group that our clients find helpful.* [partnership]
    *Karina, **I cannot take another late case** this week. **I'd be happy to work with you** to develop a schedule for staying late to address this ahead of the next time.* [partnership]

2. **Empathize, partner, and support your client or colleague.**

> *Mrs. Sangweni, I appreciate this is a **trying time** for you and Peaches.* [empathy]
>
> *It is a pleasure **to work with** you and Peaches.* [partnership]
>
> *I want to be a **team player** and be there **for you**, Karina.* [partnership]

3. **Seek your client's or colleague's perspective.**

> *Mrs. Sangweni, **who** else can sit with you and Peaches to be another set of eyes and ears?* [open-ended inquiry]
>
> *Karina, I am feeling stretched. **How** do you think we can share late appointments?* [open-ended inquiry]
>
> *Dr. Macaluso, I am handling more of the difficult client communication cases, which often results in staying late. **What** are your thoughts on how to address this?* [open-ended inquiry]

4. **Summarize and strategize.**

> *Dr. Macaluso, **in summary**, I enjoy supporting Mrs. Sangweni and Peaches, and I am concerned that my children are being neglected. I feel as if I am doing neither job well, as a veterinary technician or a mother.* [end summary]
>
> ***I suggest that** Karina and I share the late-night cases, so that it is not so hard on either of us. With your support, I will work with Karina in developing the new schedule.* [contracts for next steps]
>
> ***How** does that sound to you?* [final check]

Motivate Colleagues

Set the Scene: It is a busy day for Dr. Pompey, with five appointments in the past hour, and stress levels are rising among the veterinary team. The examination rooms were not cleaned between clients, and supplies appear scarce. The fourth client is still waiting to check out at the front desk. Frustration is growing, and patience is wearing thin! This requires a conversation with the client service coordinator, Amelia, who is on duty at the reception desk today.

It is easy to "react" versus "respond". Instead of getting angry with the team member who is causing the setbacks and delays, take a breath and dig deep. Many reasons underlie an individual's job performance, such as lack of knowledge or required skill, compassion fatigue or burnout, or life stressors (Hunter and Shaw 2015b). Assess the situation, identify the contributing factors, and use the opportunity to engage and motivate a colleague (Sidebars 10.19 and 10.20).

Sidebar 10.19   Communication Skills to Motivate Colleagues

Open-ended inquiry

Asking permission

Empathy

Partnership

End summary

Contracts for next steps

Final check

Sidebar 10.20 Essential Steps to Motivate Colleagues

To motivate colleagues: check in first, avoid making assumptions, provide support, be flexible, and follow through on the mutual plan.

1. Seek out your colleague's perspective.
2. Empathize, partner, and support your colleague.
3. Summarize and strategize.
4. Follow up and check in regularly.

1. **Seek out your colleague's perspective.**

   *I saw that the examination rooms are not ready for the next client. **How** are you doing attending to rooms between clients?* [open-ended inquiry]

   ***Could you** get the examination room ready for the next client and patient, and can we set aside some time to talk more this afternoon about balancing job responsibilities?* [asking permission]

   *Thanks for meeting. It seems like it's been **challenging** to change over examination rooms between clients.* [empathy] ***Would you like to share** with me what is going on?* [asking permission]

   ***What** else do you think is contributing?* [open-ended inquiry]

2. **Empathize, partner, and support your colleague.**

   *Our appointment schedule has been **busy**; it's **hard** to keep up with multiple doctors and rooms.* [empathy]

   *That is **a lot of life changes** to manage, and I appreciate that it is **difficult** to adjust to being the primary caregiver at home.* [empathy]

   *How can I **support you** in meeting your job and home responsibilities?* [partnership]

3. **Summarize and strategize.**

   ***It sounds like** with your recent divorce and chauffeuring the kids between two homes, it's been **exhausting**,* [empathy] *and you are struggling to focus at work.* [end summary]

   ***We** decided upon a later start time* [partnership]*, so you have transition time between dropping the kids off at school and starting your workday.* [contracts for next steps]

   ***What** other assistance do you need?* [final check]

4. **Follow up and check in regularly.**

   *I want to check in to see **how** things are going with the new schedule.* [open-ended inquiry]

   ***How** is the later start time working for you?* [open-ended inquiry]

   ***What** adjustments do **we** [partnership] need to make?* [open-ended inquiry]

Create a Toxic-Free Practice

Set the Scene: Darian is a veterinary technician with a bleeding heart for his clients and patients. In doing what Darian believes is the right thing to support clients, he stretches the practice protocols and regularly goes against doctor recommendations. This was brought to Dr. Kotchova's attention by a confused client who received differing guidance. Dr. Kotchova addresses the impact of the mixed messaging with Darian.

Toxic team attitudes include disrespect, resistance to change, lack of motivation, conflict avoidance, chronic negativity, and a desire to be the go-to person (Moore et al. 2015). Such mindsets reduce team performance and decrease job satisfaction. Toxic environments grow and form when individual toxic attitudes are contagious to other team members. Toxicity persists due to not communicating expectations, ignoring incivility, and sending mixed messages about workplace roles. To create a toxic-free practice, conduct frequent, open communication that promotes and supports a team approach to sharing the workload (Sidebars 10.21 and 10.22) (Shaw and Hunter 2016).

Sidebar 10.21   Communication Skills to Create a Toxic-Free Practice

Open-ended inquiry

Signpost

Asking permission

Chunk-and-check

Empathy

Partnership

End summary

Contracts for next steps

Final check

Sidebar 10.22   Essential Steps to Create a Toxic-Free Practice

To create a toxic-free practice: address problems early, check in with your colleague regularly, empathize and partner with your colleague, and come up with a mutual plan moving forward.

1. Check in regularly.
2. Ask permission to discuss.
3. Share concerns immediately.
4. Empathize, partner, and support your colleague.
5. Summarize and strategize.

---

1. **Check in regularly.**

   *Good morning, Darian. I wanted to take a minute to check in with you to see **how** you feel things went with our last appointment.* [open-ended inquiry]

2. **Ask permission to discuss.**

   *The client shared their thoughts, and I'm interested in **hearing your perspective**.* [signpost] ***Would you be** open to talking about it?* [asking permission]

3. **Share concerns immediately.**

   The client's feedback was that she received mixed messages from the two of us, which left her feeling baffled. [chunk] ***What** do you recall about this exchange?* [check]

   I follow practice protocols and procedures. I am concerned when I tell clients one thing and then you tell them something completely different. [chunk] ***What** are your thoughts?* [check]

4. **Empathize, partner, and support your colleague.**

   *I noticed that you appeared **frustrated** with the outcome of our last appointment.* [empathy]
   *I'd like to **work with you** to address your concerns for our clients and patients.* [partnership]
   *I know your intentions are good, and I see your **compassion** for meeting client's financial needs.* [empathy]
   *I'd appreciate it if **we** discussed your worries beforehand so that **we can work** to address them **together**.* [partnership]

5. **Summarize and strategize.**

   ***It seems like** we both want the same thing; to provide compassionate care to our clients and patients. We were just going about it differently, resulting in puzzled clients.* [end summary]
   ***Moving forward**, we are going to discuss client requests up front and **determine together** how to best approach them.* [partnership] *I appreciate you agreeing to bring these to my attention in the future.* [contracts for next steps]
   ***How** else can I support you in our working together?* [final check]

Address Workplace Bullying

Set the Scene: The alarm blares at 6:00 a.m. and warns of another day of criticism, embarrassment, and disrespect from the boss. The practice owner, Dr. Stith is sweet as pie to clients in the examination room and a tyrant in the treatment room: yelling, pacing, and berating the team for not performing up to expectations (Hunter and Shaw 2014b). It takes veterinary technician, Jordan, every effort to get the courage up to overcome the dread, climb out of bed, and get ready for work. Today is the day to tell Pamela, the practice manager, what is going on.

To address workplace bullying, the World Small Animal Veterinary Association defined principles of veterinary collegiality, including mutual respect and trust; anti-discrimination; clear, open, and honest communication; and constructive feedback (WSAVA 2021). Fear in the workplace is amplified by a lack of organizational support and systems for reporting bullying or asking for support (Appelbaum et al. 2005). Instead, team members who are afraid to assert themselves and tell the truth may eventually respond with anger and revenge (fight) or react in a passive manner (flight) by turning inward. The consequences of workplace bullying are concerning and start with harboring resentment or experiencing depression, progress to leaving the team and/or profession, and, in some extreme cases, someone taking their own life (Bulutlar and Oz 2009). To address workplace bullying, create a safe place for colleagues to be heard, acknowledge and empathize with their experiences, and provide support and resources (Sidebars 10.23 and 10.24).

Sidebar 10.23   Communication Skills to Address Workplace Bullying

Preparation

Signpost

Open-ended inquiry

Chunk-and-check

End summary

Contracts for next steps

Final check

Sidebar 10.24   Essential Steps to Address Workplace Bullying

To address workplace bullying: advocate for yourself and team, seek resources, ask for support, and keep detailed records.

1. Prepare.
2. Provide a warning shot.
3. Ask for support.
4. Share specific, descriptive, and relevant details.
5. Summarize and strategize.

1. **Prepare.** Take a deep breath, ground yourself, review the practice policies, and gather documentation.

2. **Provide a warning shot.**
   I'd like to talk to you in confidence about a situation that is frightening me. [signpost - warning shot]
   This is difficult for me to talk about. [signpost - warning shot]

3. **Ask for support.**
   I need your support. What resources does the practice provide in this circumstance? [open-ended inquiry]
   Who else can I speak to about this issue? [open-ended inquiry]

4. **Share specific, descriptive, and relevant details.**
   I documented the details of all three interactions and will share my notes with you. [chunk]
   What further information would be helpful to you? [check]

5. **Summarize and strategize.**
   Thank you for speaking with me today. I appreciate you listening and acknowledging the serious nature of this concern, especially since it's occurred multiple times now. I'm glad you agree that it needs to be addressed immediately. [end summary]
   You'll consult your colleague in human resources for more information. We'll meet later today to finalize next steps. [contracts for next steps]
   In the meantime, what do you recommend I do if it happens again? [final check]

Take It Away

1. Carry your **communication toolbox** with you into every conversation, albeit routine or challenging, with a client or a colleague.

2. Carefully choose communication skills to **acknowledge emotion; empathize, partner, and support; seek a client's or colleague's perspective; and come up with a mutual plan**.

3. In these scenarios, many of the **same communication skills** are used to effectively manage a client or colleague dilemma (i.e. open-ended inquiry, partnership, empathy, asking permission, signpost, chunk-and-check, end summary, contracts for next steps, and final check).

References

Allen, E. and Shaw, J.R. (2010). Delivering bad news: A crucial conversation. *Exceptional Veterinary Team* (January): 17–19.

Allen, E. and Shaw, J.R. (2011). The Manual: Dealing with a medical mistake. *Exceptional Veterinary Team* (March/April): 4–8.

Appelbaum, S.H., Deguire, K.J., and Lay, M. (2005). The relationship of ethical climate to deviant workplace behavior. *Corp. Gov.* 5 (4): 43–55.

Ashforth, B.E., Kreiner, G.E., and Fugate, M. (2000). All in a day's work: Boundaries and micro role transitions. *Acad. Manage. Rev.* 25 (3): 472–491.

Bensimon, E.M., Dowd, A.C., and Witham, K. (2016). Five principles for enacting equity by design. *Diversity and Democracy* 19 (1): 1–8.

Benson, K. Accessed 2023. The Anger Iceberg. Gottman Institute. https://www.gottman.com/blog/the-anger-iceberg/

Buckman, R. (1992). *How to Break Bad News: A Guide for Health Care Professionals.* Baltimore, MD: Johns Hopkins University Press.

Bulutlar, F. and Oz, E. (2009). The effects of ethical climates on bullying behavior in the workplace. *J. Bus. Eth.* 86 (3): 273–294.

Coe, J.B., Adams, C.L., and Bonnett, B.N. (2007). A focus group study of veterinarians' and pet owners' perceptions of the monetary aspects of veterinary care. *J. Am. Vet. Med. Assoc.* 231 (10): 1510–1518. https://doi.org/10.2460/javma.231.10.1510.

Criminal Watch Dog. Accessed 2023. Why you Need to Set Boundaries at Work and How to Do It. https://www.criminalwatchdog.com/resources/skill-development/setting-boundaries-at-work/

Denboba, D. (1993). MCHB/DSCSHCN Guidance for Competitive Applications, Maternal and Child Health Improvement Projects for Children with Special Health Care Needs. U.S. Department of Health and Human Services, Health Services and Resources Administration.

Hunter, L.J. and Shaw, J.R. (2014a). We need to talk: Tackling tough topics. *Veterinary Team Brief* (July): 45–46.

Hunter, L.J. and Shaw, J.R. (2014b). Fighting fear in the workplace. *Veterinary Team Brief* (July): https://www.cliniciansbrief.com/article/fighting-fear-workplace.

Hunter, L.J. and Shaw, J.R. (2015a). How to help clients angry with grief. *Clinicians Brief* (February): https://www.cliniciansbrief.com/article/how-help-clients-angry-grief.

Hunter, L.J. and Shaw, J.R. (2015b). The unmotivated team member: What is lacking? *Veterinary Team Brief* (March): 10–12.

Hunter, L.J. and Shaw, J.R. (2016). Raising awareness of diversity. *Veterinary Team Brief* (March): 27–28.

Hunter, L.J. and Shaw, J.R. (2018). Practical Tips for Talking about Money. *Clinicians Brief* (May).

Lagoni, L., Butler, C., Hetts, S. (1994). *The Human-Animal Bond and Grief.* Philadelphia, PA, WB Saunders.

Matte, A., Khosa, D., Coe, J., and Meehan, M. (2019). Impacts of the process and decision-making around companion animal euthanasia on veterinary wellbeing. *Vet. Rec.* 185 (15): 480. https://doi.org/10.1136/vr.105540.

Matte, A., Khosa, D., Coe, J. et al. (2020). Exploring pet owners' experiences and self-reported satisfaction and grief following companion animal euthanasia. *Vet. Rec.* 187 (12): e122. https://doi.org/10.1136/vr.105734.

Moore, I.C., Coe, J.B., Adams, C.L. et al. (2015). Exploring the impact of toxic attitudes and a toxic environment on the veterinary healthcare team. *Front. Vet. Sci.* 2: 1–9. https://doi.org/10.3389/fvets.2015.00078.

Patterson, K., Grenny, J., and McMillan, S. (2012). *Crucial Conversations: Tools for Talking When the Stakes Are High*. New York, NY: McGraw Hill.

Shaw, J.R., Allen, E., and Moellenberg, D.R. (2009/2010). How to discuss euthanasia with your clients. *British Small Animal Veterinary Association Student Companion*. 14–16.

Shaw, J.R. and Hunter, L.J. (2015a). Matures and millennials: Mutual goals can build mutual respect. *Veterinary Team Brief* (January/February): 54.

Shaw, J.R. and Hunter, L.J. (2015b). Setting boundaries with managers, team members, and clients. *Veterinary Team Brief* (April): 61–63.

Shaw, J.R. and Hunter, L.J. (2016). Creating a toxic-free practice environment. *Veterinary Team Brief* (October): 13–16.

US Department of Housing and Urban Development. (2023). Diversity and inclusion definitions. https://www.hud.gov/program_offices/administration/admabout/diversity_inclusion/definitions#diversity (accessed 27 November 2023).

WSAVA/FECAVA. (2021). Global principles of veterinary collegiality. https://wsava.org/wp-content/uploads/2021/02/Global-Principles-of-Veterinary-Collegiality_WSAVA-and-FECAVA.pdf (accessed 27 November 2023).

11

Now What?

Abstract

It is one task to know what the communication skills are, and it is a completely different accomplishment to implement the skills. And it is yet another achievement to correctly read a client's or colleague's nonverbal cues, be present, listen closely, and choose the appropriate communication skill at the right time and place in the conversation. From personal experience, we know that old habits die hard. Mastery comes from regular and purposeful practice. It takes time to let go of old habits and build new ones through personal commitment, discipline, and motivation. There is no ceiling to teaching and learning communication; set the course for mastery now. In this chapter, we provide 12 recommendations for how to go beyond what we shared in this book to achieve that next level by identifying goals, putting the structures in place, and rallying a support team to make it happen.

> *"The bridge between knowledge and skill is practice. The bridge between skill and mastery is time."*
>
> – Jim Bouchard

You read this book and practiced many of the exercises, and communication is now at the forefront of your mind. Where to from here? Well, a start is to return to any of the learning activities you skipped on the first read through this book. It is one task to know what the communication skills are, and it is a completely different accomplishment to implement the skills. And it is yet another achievement to correctly read a client's or colleague's nonverbal cues, be present, listen closely, and choose the appropriate communication skill at the right time and place in the conversation.

From personal experience, we know that old habits die hard. Mastery comes from regular and purposeful practice. The good news is that we are all capable of change; the bad news is that long-term habits are entrenched. Whether smoking cessation, regular exercise routines, or weight-loss programs, change is hard work and requires focused attention and motivation. It is likewise a struggle to shift from closed to open-ended inquiry, seek empathic opportunities, and converse with rather than lecture clients; these are difficult habits to break.

It takes time to let go of old habits and build new ones through personal commitment, discipline, and motivation. For new behaviors to become automatic, it takes as little as 18 days or as long as 254 days, and on average 66 days (Lally et al. 2009). Initially, developing a new skill requires effort and great concentration. Over time, it occurs unconsciously – we just do it

Developing Communication Skills for Veterinary Practice, First Edition. Jane R. Shaw and Jason B. Coe.
© 2024 John Wiley & Sons, Inc. Published 2024 by John Wiley & Sons, Inc.

without thinking about it or often realizing it (Revisit Figure 1.1 in Chapter 1). And consistent repetition hastens automaticity.

It is an infinite journey to reach effective communication. Despite advanced study, countless hours teaching others, and entire careers devoted to communication, we struggle with being good communicators all of the time. As the saying goes, "lessons are learned the hard way," and what is shared in this book comes from our own mistakes, our own paths of growth and development, and the feedback, mentorship, and coaching we received from others.

Twelve Recommendations

There is no ceiling on teaching and learning communication; set the course for mastery now. Identify your goals, put the structure in place, and rally your support team to make it happen. Here are our **12 recommendations** for how to go beyond what we shared in this book:

1. **Begin with yourself.** Develop your own communication toolbox initially by building competence and confidence over time. Facing these personal struggles and challenges fosters a more patient and compassionate approach to mentoring colleagues. Note and share your success stories, including what is different, what worked, and what results you achieved. And be vulnerable in sharing challenges, and acknowledge the difficulties, hardships, and struggles that get in the way.

2. **Identify personal sources of motivation.** It is easier to kick habits that align with our personal values than from external pressure of others. We each possess a unique "why" that motivates us, which becomes a personal mantra to lead change forward. The stronger the reasons for change, the quicker and more robust the progress.
   Here are some guiding questions:
   a. What is driving you to want to change the way you communicate?
   b. What difference will it make in your day-to-day?
   c. How will it help you achieve your personal or professional goals?
   d. How will it impact your relationships with yourself, clients, and colleagues?

3. **Be accountable.** Balance being your best friend and guide, cheerleader and critic, and optimist and pessimist. Listen to your inner stories – are they messages of triumph or defeat? Set goals, record progress, check in regularly, and modify the approach as necessary.

4. **Seek support.** Compile a team of friends and family, colleagues and supervisors, and a professional counselor or coach. The support team's role is both on the sidelines cheering with words of encouragement (easy part) and assisting you in seeing your blind spots and taking an honest look at yourself (hard part). This entails seeking out and being receptive to specific, descriptive, and constructive feedback.

5. **Choose specific, manageable, and bite-size daily goals.** Choose one of the communication skills to work on at a time. Start with the skills that need polishing and sharpening, and then tackle those that require development from the ground up. Effective learning happens under a degree of tension and requires embracing awkwardness and discomfort. Find the "just right" amount of challenge within your personal limits.

6. **Expect progress to wax and wane.** Sometimes change feels like it is going gangbusters and at other times like dragging feet. On hard days, be patient and forgiving, keep your mantra in mind, and check in with your support team. On good days, mark milestones and celebrate accomplishments. Either way, reaffirm your commitment.

7. **Share with colleagues.** Revisit Chapter 9 on communication coaching for this step. Start with one-on-one coaching sessions with colleagues, and grow to offering team training sessions. At the start, tackle more routine communication tasks, such as agenda-setting, information-gathering, or team meetings, and then move to more challenging conversations such as delivering bad news, conflict management, financial discussions, or disclosing medical errors.

8. **Build a communication team**. To enhance sustainability, form a group of internal communication gurus to serve as train-the-trainers in the practice. It takes a village to support an entire practice team and shift the communication culture. These individuals serve as colleague coaches and mentors and assist with developing a training program.

9. **Select for communication during hiring.** Look at your interviewing techniques when hiring a new team member. Review the questions to determine if they are phrased as closed- or open-ended inquiries. Employ behavioral interviewing, and offer working interviews to see potential colleagues' communication in action. Assess their receptivity to feedback and coaching and willingness to grow and develop. Seek new colleagues with growth versus fixed mindsets.

10. **Incorporate communication training in the onboarding process**. Include communication skill development as one of the key tasks when onboarding new colleagues. Create individual professional development plans for enhancing communication skills in their practice role. Develop their communication skills through observation, coaching, feedback, and role-play.

11. **Be diligent, flexible, and patient with others**. For as long as it takes for someone to develop a new habit, they need mentorship, guidance, and support from their supervisor and colleagues. Establish a routine for regular check-ins, progress reports, and debriefings, and adjust the plan accordingly. Balance goal-setting with recognizing achievements and progress.

12. **Make communication your practice culture.** Embrace communication as a core practice value embedded through each conversation. Set an intention to be purposeful communicators. This means walking the talk, welcoming change, and supporting growth. There is no ceiling on effective communication, and as human beings, we will never be perfect. Recognize when good communication is happening, perceive your abilities and limits, and make a recovery or identify learning or teaching moments when conversations go awry.

Put the Communication Skills into Practice

We provide two final capstone exercises for your journey toward mastery: one to prepare for a challenging conversation with a client or colleague and the other to conduct communication or video-review rounds with the practice team.

Do-It-Yourself Exercise

Exercise 11.1   Challenging Conversations (Adapted from American Association of American Medical Colleges, 2023 with permission)
A challenging conversation is one in which the stakes and consequences are high for client, patient, colleague, or self. Since parties are deeply invested in these discussions, emotions run strong, and with opposing viewpoints, there is the potential for disagreement (Patterson et al. 2011). Due to the intensity, it is easy to talk too much; and with blood pounding in our ears, it may be difficult to listen. When emotionally triggered, we tend to interrupt others; get angry, confused, or derailed; or lose track of what we would like to say or our end goal.

It is easy for the conversation to go off the rails, especially with multiple passionate individuals with diverse opinions and unpredictable responses. The conversation quickly stalls or turns into a venting session and does not move toward a constructive resolution. With the potential for volatility, invest in preparing ahead of time to stay on course, ground your emotions, and prevent verbal diarrhea. A plan is necessary to be present, center yourself, and be proactive in facilitating these challenging discussions.

There are **four steps** to this exercise:

1. Reflect on a struggle with a client or colleague through journaling. Take a deep dive, view the situation from other's perspective, be accountable for your role, and consider the consequences.

2. Compose an opening statement. This is an outline for how you will enter the conversation and get it off to a strong start.

3. Role-play and practice ahead of time with a trusted colleague. Try out your opening statement live with a colleague, coach, or friend. Request their specific descriptive, balanced and relevant feedback and revise the statement as needed.

4. Deliver your opening statement to the intended client or colleague.

We provide guiding questions, suggested skills, and structured outlines for each step below.

Step 1: Journal about the Situation

Be brave, open, and honest with yourself, look deep inside, and take accountability for your role in this issue. This exercise may be difficult, and you may need to work through emotional triggers to be objective. It is easy to be the victim when we feel hurt or wronged. Viewing the greater impact on others invites us to get outside of ourselves to be creative in moving toward partnership and solution.

1. Reflect on a potential upcoming conversation with client(s) or colleague(s). Choose one person with whom you have an unresolved issue(s).

2. Clarify the issue.
   a. What is going on? Provide specific examples.
   b. How long has it been going on?
   c. How bad is it?
   d. What are the indicators of a stressed relationship?

3. Determine the impact:
   a. What is the impact on you?
   b. What is the impact on your patient, client, colleague, or team?
   c. What is the impact on practice work processes, values, or culture?
   d. What is at stake if it continues?

4. What is your contribution to this issue? Dig deep – tell yourself the truth!

5. Describe the ideal outcome. By resolving this issue, what difference will it make? What will be the benefits to patients, clients, colleagues, the team, or yourself?

Step 2: Compose an Opening Statement (One to Two Minutes in Length)

Your opening statement is intended to engage the other party, put them at ease, start building rapport, and state your purpose. Respond to each prompt with one short and simple sentence to prevent turning it into a lecture and losing the other person's attention. This is just the beginning; if done well, there will be an opportunity to share more as the conversation evolves.

1. Offer an empathic or reflective listening statement to name the issue/concern.

2. Select a specific observable example that illustrates the challenging behavior or situation, and describe its impact on your patient, client, colleague, team, or yourself?

   When I saw or I heard (behavior), the impact for me was (self-disclosure).

3. Identify your contribution to the problem.

4. Indicate your commitment to resolving the issue.

5. Pose an open-ended question to explore the other person's perspective and pause to invite your client or colleague to respond.

Step 3: Role-Play and Practice

Before delivering your opening statement, set up a dress rehearsal to try it with a trusted colleague or friend. Choose someone who will be direct, honest, and supportive in their feedback. It is best if they are knowledgeable and aware of the communication skills and even more so if they are highly observant and attentive to details.

1. **Brief your partner.** Share with your colleague, coach, or friend a brief three-sentence verbal description of the issue. This is a good readiness test. If you boil the problem down to its essential ingredients, it is a sign that you worked through the situation yourself. If it turns into a lecture, it means there is more personal work to be done before engaging in the challenging conversation.

2. **Share their perspective.** Provide a short characterization of the client or colleague in the troublesome situation so your trusted colleague, coach, or friend takes on their perspective during the role-play. This will aid them in determining how the opening statement might be received.

3. **Ask for confidentiality.** Ask your colleague, coach, or friend to ensure that this is a safe, supportive, and confidential learning space and that this conversation will not be shared with others.

4. **Request feedback.** Ask your colleague, coach, or friend to provide specific feedback, including perceived strengths and areas for development. Request suggestions and examples for how to strengthen the opening statement, including both verbal and nonverbal communication skills.

5. **Practice the opening statement.** Deliver the opening statement to your colleague, coach, or friend as authentically as possible, as if they were the intended audience.

6. **Invite feedback.** Listen to the feedback with an open mind and heart. Ask for clarification and specific suggestions as needed.

7. **Edit the opening statement.** Revise the opening statement based on the feedback received as needed.

Step 4: Schedule the Meeting with Your Client or Colleague

It's time to deliver the opening statement for real. Trust that the thoughtful and diligent preparation invested will pay off. Know that it will not be perfect, we all make mistakes, and it is likely you will wish you had said or done something differently. It is important to step out of self-critique and focus on your courageous intent to lead this challenging conversation. With each crucial conversation under your belt, you will become more confident and competent the next time around.

Engage-the-Entire-Team Exercise

Exercise 11.2   Communication or Video-Review Rounds
Veterinary professionals are familiar with the format of clinical case rounds in which the team briefs each other on cases in the hospital, providing updates and outlining treatment plans. As the team walks from cage to cage, a colleague presents their case. The veterinary professionals discuss case management to capitalize on shared knowledge. It is a method of ensuring continuity of care and sharing best practices between veterinary team members to enhance patient care and reduce medical errors.

Likewise, the purpose of communication rounds is to take time to reflect on interactions with clients or between team members to enhance client care, quality of service, teamwork, and morale. Cases are presented either from memory or via a video recording (preferred) of an actual client or colleague interaction. Such dialogue fosters skill acquisition, open communication, role-modeling, and an opportunity for feedback and support of team members.

Communication rounds capitalize on the collective wisdom of the practice team. The coach does just that: they are someone who listens, poses questions, and cultivates conversation, instead of provides answers. An **effective coach utilizes a partner approach** and recognizes the group's or individual's expertise, compared to an expert who directs the conversation. The goal is to engage the individual or as many colleagues as possible in the discussion. Consider rotating the coaching role among the team so everyone develops this skillset.

The coach asks questions, fosters discussion, elicits contributions from the group, and summarizes key points. Although coaches offer input and make suggestions, it is often more meaningful to do so after obtaining input from the team – and even then, only if it adds something new to the discussion. The greatest challenge as a coach is to keep your mouth shut and let the group do the work.

There are **four steps** to conduct communication or video-review rounds:

1. Establish small-group guidelines with the team.

2. Commit to a regular schedule of communication or video-review rounds.

3. Prepare the team ahead of time by identifying communication skill(s) objectives and either choosing a case to present or a video recording of a client or colleague interaction.

4. Conduct the communication or video-review rounds session.

We provide guiding questions, suggested skills, and structured outlines for each step below.

Step 1: Establish Small-Group Guidelines

The goal of communication rounds is ongoing professional development in a supportive environment. A safe space allows individuals to be vulnerable, receptive to feedback, and open to alternative approaches. Safety is a prerequisite for colleagues to share case interactions or video recordings and seek valued input from others. In communication rounds, we establish a judgment-free zone where there is no right or wrong and the intention is to swap trade secrets for communicating with clients and colleagues.

A good starting place to create a constructive learning environment is to establish group guidelines. These are behavioral norms defined by the team; they promote a safe and comfortable learning environment that balances providing support with fostering growth and skill development. Guiding questions are provided in Box 11.1 to prime the group's thinking. Find sample small-group guidelines in Box 9.6 in Chapter 9.

Box 11.1   Guiding Questions to Establish Small-Group Guidelines

What makes you feel comfortable sharing and hearing from the group?
What helps you to share with others?
What support would you like from the group?
What opens you up to receiving feedback?
How do you like to hear suggestions?

Step 2: Commit to a Regular Schedule

Set a goal to conduct communication rounds every 2 weeks for an average of 30 minutes to an hour. Even rounds as short as 20 minutes are productive and keep communication skills in everyone's minds. Using the format given here, it is possible to review five colleagues' case scenarios or video recordings (2–3 minutes each) in an hour. Doing so requires setting the agenda, sticking to the timeline, keeping feedback succinct, and being attentive to the structure.

Step 3: Prepare the Team ahead of Time

1. **Identify communication skill(s) objectives.**
   Ask everyone to identify the communication skill(s) they are working on. Use the content of this book, which is based on the logical flow and sections of a clinical interview and 20 core communication skills. A shared learning culture enhances the efficacy of skill acquisition when everyone is talking about and working on similar communication skills.

2. **Choose a case scenario, or video-record a client or colleague interaction.**
   Colleagues choose between re-creating an interaction from memory or presenting an audio or video recording of a client or colleague interaction. An audio or video recording is preferred if the practice possesses the capability, as it captures both verbal and nonverbal communication. A two- to three-minute video-recorded interaction provides enough material to work with. Ensure that colleagues mark the time stamp or save a short clip of the video segment ahead of time. Otherwise, ask colleagues to reflect on a recent interaction

they might like to share and identify a specific part of the conversation to present to the group. It is equally beneficial to view a successful exchange, as one that was challenging, to reinforce what worked.

Step 4: Conduct the Communication or Video-Review Rounds

Following is a conversational model that provides a tool for coaches; we walk through each step and provide guiding coaching questions. It is perfectly acceptable the first few times to read verbatim from the outline and example questions; that is why we provide them here.

1. Set the Scene for Rounds (five minutes):

> **Coach:** *The purpose of communication rounds is to set aside time every other week to reflect on interactions with our clients and colleagues. This presents an opportunity to discuss communication situations that you found challenging to seek support and guidance, or a successful communication scenario to celebrate. Let me remind you of the group guidelines we created so that we all feel safe to share.*

2. Conduct the rounds (50 minutes [5 colleagues, 10 minutes each]): Repeat the following steps for each volunteer.

   a. **Select a volunteer to present a case or to view their video recording.**
   Who would like to start us off by sharing a recent client or colleague interaction or an audio or video recording?

   b. **Brief the volunteer.**
      i. *What communication skill(s) were you working on?*
      ii. *Briefly share with us the background of this scenario.*
      iii. *What led you to share this interaction with us?*
      iv. *Now, what feedback from us would be most helpful to you?*

   c. **Prepare peers for feedback.**
   Prepare the peers to take notes and capture specific examples. Focus peers on observing the communication skill(s) their colleague is working on and/or skills highlighted in their request for feedback. While listening to the case review or watching the audio or video, ask that peers record verbatim examples of what their colleague said (verbal communication) or a detailed description of what they did (nonverbal communication).

   When developing your feedback, I'd like to request two sentences from each observer:

      i. *Your favorite quote of the communication skill your colleague was working on (e.g. open-ended inquiry)*
         a. *In this example, record your favorite open-ended inquiry.*
      ii. *An alternative of how you would use that communication skill in this scenario.*
         b. *What is an open-ended inquiry you might ask, or how might you rephrase one of the closed-ended inquiries?*

   d. **Listen to the case or watch the audio or video recording** (two- to three-minute segment per participant).

e. **Debrief.**

    i. Volunteer self-assessment: *What was it like to watch it again? What did you see or hear?*

    ii. Volunteer check-in: *Would you like to hear your colleagues' thoughts?*

    iii. Invite peer feedback: *What was your favorite example of an open-ended inquiry? How would you use open-ended inquiry in this scenario?*

    iv. Volunteer rewind: *Of the suggestions, what would you like to role-play and practice?*

    v. Volunteer take-away: *What is your aha moment? What is a key lesson? What is resonating with you?*

Close the rounds (five minutes)

To close the session, request a lesson learned and a next step from everyone.
What communication skill(s) are you working on moving forward?
What will you do differently in your next client or colleague interaction?

Take It Away

1. **Mastery** is embracing learning and continuously taking communication skills to the next level. It is a long, windy, and worthy path with no clear endpoint.

2. Hold a clear vision, set realistic milestones, and maintain a **growth mindset**; that is what we ask of ourselves and our colleagues.

3. What we put into it is what we will receive in return, making a difference in the lives of our patients, clients, colleagues, and ourselves – truly **meaningful work**.

References

Lally, P., van Jaarsveld, C.H.M., Potts, H.W.W., and Wardle, J. (2009). How are habits formed: Modelling habit formation in the real world. *Eur. J. Soc. Psychol.* 40: 998–1009. https://doi.org/10.1002/ejsp.674.

Patterson, K., Grenny, J., McMillan, R., and Switzler, A. (2011). *Crucial Conversation Tools for Talking when the Stakes Are High*. New York, NY: McGraw-Hill.

Association of American Medical Colleges (2023). *Leading organizations to health*. https://www.aamc.org/career-development/leadership-development/leading-organizations-health (accessed 28 November 2023).

Appendices – Tools to Support Coaching and Communication Skills Learning Sessions

A. **20 communication skills** – This is an easy-to-reference handout with a list of the 20 communication skills introduced throughout the book, including definitions and examples. This format is portable to take to communication learning sessions for ready access and clarification. It is also a helpful resource for choosing individual or group communication goals prior to a learning session.

B. **Coach process card** – This is a step-by-step guide for a communication coach to lead a one-on-one or group communication learning session. For a novice coach, this script outlines the steps of communication coaching and is a well-worn tool of seasoned coaches. Literally walk through each step and choose from suggested questions and phrases. Trust that over time, you'll make the script your own and improvise and discover wording that fits you best. Lean on the communication coaching process and structure because it creates a strong foundation for establishing a safe and supportive learning environment.

C. **Communication skills checklist** – This is a form for coaches and colleagues to capture detailed notes during an individual or group communication learning activity (e.g. role-play, colleague observation). Best feedback practices include providing specific, detailed, balanced, and relevant behavioral descriptions. This template is designed to capture well-executed examples of the communication skills, as well as suggestions of questions or statements to try. Focus on capturing notes about two or three communication goals your colleague is working on. Write down your favorite quotes of the skills, and propose new ideas for phrases to experiment with.

Developing Communication Skills for Veterinary Practice, First Edition. Jane R. Shaw and Jason B. Coe.
© 2024 John Wiley & Sons, Inc. Published 2024 by John Wiley & Sons, Inc.

Appendix A

20 Communication Skills

Skill	Definition	Example
	Opening-the-Interaction	
Preparation	Take time to prepare for the interaction.	Review the medical record. Take a breath/break. Reflect on the scenario.
Introduction	Create a warm welcome and initial rapport: 1. Make an introduction to the client(s) (or colleague) and clarify your role. 2. Make an introduction to the pet(s). 3. Invite the client(s) (or colleague) to introduce themselves and their pet(s). 4. Demonstrate interest in the client(s) (or colleague) and their pet(s). 5. Address any immediate concern(s) right away.	*Hello, my name is Brad, I am a veterinary technician, I use he/him/his pronouns, and I will be taking care of you and Sasha today.* *Hi Sasha, pretty girl! Come on out of your crate when you're ready.* *How would you like to be addressed? It's nice to meet you, Mrs. Kittredge.* *I see that this is your second visit here with Sasha. You saw Dr. Rodriguez last time and are scheduled today to see Dr. Hammond.* *What do you or Sasha need while you wait for Dr. Hammond?*

Agenda-setting	Identify the client's (colleague's) full agenda:
	
	1. Elicit your client's (or colleague's) agenda:
	  a. Reason(s) for the visit or meeting
	  b. Client (colleague) concerns
	  c. Goals, expectations, and priorities
	2. Summarize the client's (or colleague's) agenda.
	3. Check for remaining items.
	4. Offer your (i.e., the veterinary professional's) agenda items.
	5. Negotiate a mutual agenda.
	6. Summarize the mutually agreed-on agenda.
		What brings you and Sasha in today?
		What other concerns do you have with Sasha?
		What goals do you have for today's appointment?
		What are you hoping we can do for you and Sasha today?
		What you'd like to do today is Sasha's physical examination, update her vaccinations, trim her nails, and talk about her biting behavior.
		Of the items on your list, what's your number-one priority for our visit today?
		What else would you like to discuss?
		I'd like to talk to you about Sasha's dental care and weight management as well today. Would that be all right with you?
		So, our plan includes Sasha's physical exam and vaccinations, nail trim, biting behavior, dental care, and weight management discussions.

Developing Communication Skills for Veterinary Practice, First Edition. Jane R. Shaw and Jason B. Coe.
© 2024 John Wiley & Sons, Inc. Published 2024 by John Wiley & Sons, Inc.

Skill	Definition	Example
Information-Gathering		
Open-ended inquiry	Invite your client (or colleague) to tell their story, introduce the topic, and start with a broad exploration.	*Describe for me how Sasha has been doing since we saw her a year ago.*
Closed-ended inquiry	Gather key details or confirm, clarify, or correct information.	*So, when did Sasha's biting behavior start?*
Pause	Allow space between taking turns speaking, and be mindful of interrupting or cutting off your client (colleague). Use silence to create time for your client (colleague) to examine their thoughts and feelings.	Take a breath. Wait for a client cue. Count to 3.
Minimal encouragers	Use small words that invite your client (colleague) to continue speaking.	*Uh huh, um-hum, go on, yes, yeah, oh, wow, really, I see*
Reflective listening	Ensure that your client (colleague) has been heard, and invite correction, clarification, or addition to the story. Take stock of what you learned and what else you'd like to know.	*It seems like her biting behavior is causing a problem for all of you.*
Attending to Relationships		
Nonverbal behaviors	Display physical expressions that accompany language use:	
	1. Kinesics	Attentive body posture, calm body movements, expressive gestures, good eye contact, self-managed responses
	2. Proxemics	Appropriate distance from the client, turning toward the client, sitting at the same level as the client
	3. Paralanguage	Confident voice tone, appropriate volume, comfortable pacing
	4. Autonomic responses	Tearing up, flushing, and sweating
	5. Environmental cues	Professional appearance and welcoming hospital setting
Empathy	Communicate your understanding of the emotional state of your client (colleague). Acknowledge, validate, and normalize their emotional response.	*I see how much you love Sasha and how much this biting behavior is distressing you and making it difficult for you to interact with her.*
Partnership	Express the desire to work together toward a mutual goal, and inform your client (or colleague) that they are not alone and will be supported along the way.	*We'll work together to get to the bottom of this biting behavior.*
Asking permission	Checks to see if your client (or colleague) is ready or if they will give consent to move forward in the conversation, procedure, agenda, or decision.	*Would it be all right if we sat down and I asked you some questions about Sasha's behavior?*

(Continued)

Skill	Definition	Example
Attending to Tasks		
Logical sequence	Progress through the clinical interview or meeting in a logical order: 1. Opening-the-interaction 2. Information-gathering 3. Physical examination 4. Diagnostic and treatment planning 5. Closing-the-interaction	Take a stepwise approach to the clinical interview or meeting, and do not move ahead or skip steps. Balance attending to relationships and tasks.
Signpost	Use transitional statements to mark where the conversation has been and/or where it is going next.	*There are three options to address Sasha's behavior that I would like to discuss with you.*
Internal summary	Recap your client's (or colleague's) agenda, information gathered, or diagnostic or treatment plan and enable clients (or colleagues) to review and clarify information prior to moving on in the clinical interview or meeting.	*It sounds like Sasha is fitting well into your lives and that she is healthy. You love her very much, but she's been a nuisance lately, biting members of the household. Your priority is to spend our time together today addressing her behavioral issue. If we have time, the secondary issue is updating her vaccinations. What else would you like to add?*
Diagnostic and Treatment Planning		
Easily understood language	Avoid medical jargon, unless appropriate, and instead use simple lay language, or define terminology in a manner that your client (or colleague) can comprehend.	*We can use a medication to reduce the biting behavior while you work with the behaviorist to modify Sasha's behavior for the long run.*
Chunk-and-check	Speak in small, easily understandable phrases, one to three sentences at a time. Pause or check for your client's (or colleague's) understanding before proceeding.	*You are correct that addressing Sasha's biting behavior will take time, persistence, and consistency. I'd recommend engaging with a behaviorist, who can develop protocols for responding to her biting behavior. What additional information can I provide you on this option for Sasha?*
Closing-the-Interaction		
End summary	Recap information to capture multiple pieces of data, pulling them all together and highlighting salient points to take home.	*We talked about Sasha's biting behavior and the impact on the family dynamic. Re-homing is off the table as a possible option, and you are interested in consulting a behaviorist. What would you like to add?*
Contracts for next steps	Define next steps, and outline the roles and responsibilities of both parties moving forward.	*Since discussion of Sasha's biting behavior was paramount today, we agreed to schedule a recheck examination to update her vaccinations. I will do her nail trim shortly. And send you home with contact information for a veterinary behaviorist.*
Final check	Offer a final check at the close to ensure that all questions and concerns have been fully addressed and understood.	*As we close our visit, what remaining questions do you have?*

Adapted from Communication Skills Checklist, Jane R. Shaw, DVM, PhD, (2023). Communication Curriculum, Veterinary Communication for Professional Excellence. Fort Collins, CO: Colorado State University.

Appendix B

Coaching Process Card

Open-the-Session

Establish rapport	*Thanks for inviting me to join you!* *How are you feeling about this interaction/appointment?*
Demonstrate interest and concern	*You may feel nervous or awkward being observed.* *Thank you ahead of time for being open-minded and trying new approaches.*
Purpose of the interaction/ appointment	*The purpose is to support you to achieve your communication goals.*
Safe and supportive	*This is an opportunity to practice, not an evaluation.* *We are going to work as a team to support each other.*
Confidentiality	*Vegas rules: What happens here, stays here.*
Agenda-setting	*We will begin by talking about your communication objectives.* *Then I'll watch your interaction/appointment.* *After the interaction/appointment, we will debrief, starting with you.* *If you are open to it, I'll share some reflections for consideration.*

Prep-the-Interaction/Appointment

Refer to the Communication Skills Checklist (Appendix C)

Review the interviewer's objectives	*What skills are you working on?* *What led you to choose those skills?* *Which skill is a strength?* *Which skill is a stretch?*
Prepare for the case	*Tell me about this interaction/appointment.* *What are you walking into?* *How will you address that challenge?*

Developing Communication Skills for Veterinary Practice, First Edition. Jane R. Shaw and Jason B. Coe.
© 2024 John Wiley & Sons, Inc. Published 2024 by John Wiley & Sons, Inc.

Brainstorm communication skills and examples	*Let's brainstorm examples of your communication skills.*
	What would that sound like?
	How might you use that skill?
Plan for feedback	*What feedback would be most helpful to you?*
	What would you like me to look for?
	How can I help you with that?
Support	*What else do you need to prepare for this interaction/ appointment?*
	How can I best support you?
	What questions do you have before we start?

Observe-the-Interaction/Appointment

START RECORDING if appropriate

Introduce	Yourself to the client
Purpose	Share with the client the goals of the observation
Obtain	Client consent
Refer	Communication Skills Checklist (Appendix C)
Note	Examples of communication objectives demonstrated

Take-a-Break in the Interaction/Appointment

Coaching during a client appointment
If a natural break occurs in the appointment, check in.

Purpose	Reflect, refocus on objectives, and brainstorm new approaches.	**REMEMBER** You don't need good answers, just good questions.
Promote self-discovery	*What is the client's agenda?*	
	What did you learn from the history?	Let them discover it for themselves!
	How will you offer/negotiate a plan?	
	What have you accomplished so far?	
Create a specific plan	*What would you like to do next?*	
	How will your objectives help you achieve that?	
	What would that sound like?	

Coaching during a simulated interaction (e.g. role-play)

Purpose	Reflect, refocus objectives, and brainstorm new approaches
Promote self-discovery	*How's it going?* Or *How are you feeling?* *What else do you need to know?* *Where would you like to go next?*
Create a specific plan	*Where would you like to start?* *What are you going to say?* *How about you pick up when the client said . . .*
Rewind	When you sense an opportunity for a case reset or skill redemption, take a step back in the simulated interaction. *What would you like to try differently?* *Where would you like the client to start?* *Let's rewind to. . .*

STOP RECORDING

Timing of Breaks

Flustered at **Start**, BREAK
How are you doing?
What do you need to accomplish?

Once **Agenda** is Completed ("That's everything"), BREAK
What is the client's agenda?
How do you know you have the whole agenda?
What's the client's priority?
What will you explore first given the client's priority?

During **Information-Gathering**, BREAK
What agenda items have you addressed?
What else would you like to learn from the client?
What type of information have you gathered – patient, client, or environment?
What else are you curious about?
How are you doing at meeting your communication objectives?

Entering **Planning**, BREAK
How will you proceed into a plan, considering the client's priorities?
What's your next step?
What are some perceived barriers to the plan?
How will you overcome these barriers?
How will your objectives help you achieve that?

Debrief-the-Interaction/Appointment

Interviewer's self assessment	*Tell me about that experience.* *What did you think?* Or *How did you feel about that?* *What went well?* *What would you like to do over?*	**Phrasing Specific, Descriptive, Balanced, and Relevant Feedback**
Rewind	The purpose of rewind is to practice the skill. *Would you like to give that a try with me?* *Let's see what that sounds like.*	*My favorite quote was . . .* *The client responded well when you said . . .* *You learned critical information when you asked . . .* *What were your thoughts when . . . happened?* *One thought I had is . . .*
Coach or peer feedback	*Would you be open to feedback?* *What would you like to practice with me?* *How would you phrase that?*	*I wonder what might have happened if you had asked or said . . .* *One thing I'd try is . . .*
Wrap up the Interaction/ Appointment	*What is your takeaway from this experience?* *What would you like to work on in your next interaction/appointment?* *How will that look?*	

Close-the-Session

Identify learning plan	*What is your take-home message today?* *What was an "aha" moment for you?* *What objective(s) did you achieve?* *What would you like to do next?* *How can I support you moving forward?*

Adapted from Coaching Process Card, Jane R. Shaw, DVM, PhD, (2023). Communication Curriculum, Veterinary Communication for Professional Excellence. Fort Collins, CO: Colorado State University.

Appendix C

Communication Skills Checklist

Date:

Colleague's Name: **Coach Name:**

Scenario:

Communication Goals:

1.
2.
3.

Write skill examples and suggestions in the space provided.

OPENING-THE-INTERACTION
1. Preparation
2. Introduction
3. Agenda-setting
INFORMATION-GATHERING
4. Open-ended inquiry
5. Closed-ended inquiry
6. Pause
7. Minimal encouragers
8. Reflective listening

Developing Communication Skills for Veterinary Practice, First Edition. Jane R. Shaw and Jason B. Coe.
© 2024 John Wiley & Sons, Inc. Published 2024 by John Wiley & Sons, Inc.

ATTENDING TO RELATIONSHIPS
9. Nonverbal behaviors
10. Empathy
11. Partnership
12. Asking permission

ATTENDING TO TASKS
13. Logical sequence
14. Signpost
15. Internal summary

DIAGNOSTIC AND TREATMENT PLANNING
16. Easily understood language
17. Chunk-and-check

CLOSING-THE-INTERACTION
18. End summary
19. Contracts for next steps
20. Final check

OVERALL COMMENTS:

Source: Jane R. Shaw, DVM, PhD, (2023). Communication Curriculum, Veterinary Communication for Professional Excellence. Fort Collins, CO: Colorado State University.

Index

Note: *Italic* page numbers refer to *figure* and **Bold** page numbers reference to **tables** and page numbers followed by "b" indicates boxes

Developing Communication Skills for Veterinary Practice, First Edition. Jane R. Shaw and Jason B. Coe.
© 2024 John Wiley & Sons, Inc. Published 2024 by John Wiley & Sons, Inc.